MEDICINE IN OLD AGE

Articles published in
the *British Medical Journal*

Published by the British Medical Association
Tavistock Square, London WC1H 9JR

ISBN 0 900221 93 3

Made and printed in England by
The Devonshire Press,
Printing House, Barton Road, Torquay

PREFACE

by

Editor, *British Medical Journal*

Geriatrics is a specialty in which Britain is acknowledged to lead the world. The pioneering work of men such as Sheldon, Lord Amulree and Howell has done much to establish the presentday pattern of care in this field: full-time consultants in many district hospitals, day-hospital units, and university departments—all of which have helped to convert mere existence into a full life for many elderly patients. Moreover, the specialty is expanding, as witnessed by the recent creation of several university chairs and the publication of specialist journals devoted to ageing and the medicine of old age.

None of these developments have come a moment too soon, for as everybody recognises, the proportion of the elderly in our population will almost certainly have risen considerably by the end of the century. Nevertheless, because of the recent development of the specialty many doctors may have qualified knowing comparatively little about it, and last year to remedy this the *B.M.J.* published a series of commissioned articles in its ' Medical Practice ' section. Having been revised by their authors, these have now been collected into this book, which we hope will form a useful introduction to an important subject.

MARTIN WARE

July 1974

CONTENTS

Contents

Treatment of the
"Irremediable" Elderly Patient

BY

BERNARD ISAACS

HERE is a title as full of questions as a pomegranate is full of seeds. How does one treat the irremediable? If the irremediable is treated, is it irremediable? Is "to treat" less than "to remedy"? And why the contiguity of "irremediable" and "elderly"? Are all elderly irremediable? Are all irremediable elderly? These questions concern attitudes. They are important because attitudes rather than expertise determine the outcome of treatment.

ATTITUDES

There was a time, before I entered on that state of grace peculiar to the geriatrician, when the phrase "treatment of the irremediable elderly patient" would have concisely defined geriatrics for me. Later, when I began to work in geriatric medicine, I would have indignantly rebutted the implication that anyone or anything old was irremediable; for did we not profess our faith in the liturgical phrase: "an ill old person is ill because he is ill and not because he is old"? Now, after years of the pragmatic practice of my art, I welcome the recognition that we geriatricians, and not we alone, devote much of our activities to the treatment of the irremediable. Few diseases at any age are cured; most whisper to the patient of their continuing presence, long after the ink is dry on the discharge letter. The treatment of the irremediable is both a worthy objective and an accurate description of much modern medicine.

WHO ARE THE "IRREMEDIABLE"?

First who are they not? They are not, and must not be confounded with, the undiagnosed. They are not the confused, the incontinent, the senile. Confusion and incontinence are symptoms of impaired function of the nervous system and bladder. The words give no information on cause or cure. The term "senility" offends the geriatrician; it requires an effort of will even to write it. In my mind's eye I see the word garbed in a cloak of black, with the blood of ill old people dripping from its lanky fingers. A melodramatic image perhaps; but how often has the attachment of this label to an ill old patient spelt the end of

9

diagnostic and therapeutic endeavour, and condemned him to a slow death by stewing in his own urine?

Every ill person of whatever age has a right to a diagnosis; and only when this has been established is it possible to talk about remediability or irremediability. "Senility" is not a diagnosis; it spells relegation for the patient and abdication by the doctor. I look forward to the day when the word "senility" will have disappeared from acceptable medical terminology, as the word "insanity" has done.

IRREVERSIBLE DISEASE

Many pathological processes which are common in old age are at present irreversible. These include neoplasm, atherosclerosis, and neuronal degeneration—one or more of which accompany most old people on their last long journey to the grave. It is among these sadly disabled people that the doctor seeks opportunities for effective intervention; and opportunities abound.

TREATING THE IRREMEDIABLE

A man of 69 was seen for the first time two months after the onset of a right hemiplegia, and after failure of a trial of rehabilitation. The patient was bedfast, there was no return of movement to the affected side, he had a catheter in his bladder, and he was unable to speak or to comprehend. He had been found picking faeces from his rectum and smearing them on his locker. He disturbed other patients by shouting. He had struck out at the nurses, and given his wife a black eye.

First the wife was interviewed. Who was this man? What kind of person was he? He had been a good husband, a loving father, abstemious, a steady and conscientious worker, a keen amateur gardener, a fit man, proud of his good health and work record, inclined to disparage those less healthy than himself. What did she know of his illness? What did she say to him when she visited? She talked to him; sometimes, she thought, he understood her; sometimes he pushed her away and turned his head away from her. Once he lifted his hand to her, a thing he never did in his life. Did she ever cry? She had gone home and wept to herself every night since his illness began, but hadn't told anyone. Did she think he was going to die? She didn't know, but sometimes she found herself half-wishing that he would, and that made her feel wicked. Had she told this to anyone? Not a soul. Had anyone told her what was likely to happen to her husband? No one.

Next the patient was examined. His tongue was dry, his rectum packed with hard dry faeces. There was a pressure sore on his heel; his urine was infected; his haemoglobin level had dropped. He couldn't speak or understand language, but he could pick up situational clues. He could sing "Tipperary" with the words matching the tune; he could count up to ten if he was started off; he could correctly identify "bottle," "tumbler," "spectacles." He could build toy blocks one on top of the other. He could match dominoes. He had no movement in his arm or leg, but he could sit up in bed with minimal support. Suddenly, out of this irremediable situation, all kinds of opportunities of effective intervention were appearing, like crocuses piercing the wintry soil.

The nurses began first. They put him on a fluid chart, gave him adequate nourishing drinks, talking to him as they did so, telling him what they were trying to do, encouraging him to take the cup and drink himself, trying to find out what he would like—orange juice, milk, tea, beer, perhaps even a glass of whisky. They found his pipe, his false teeth, his razor and comb. They emptied his bowel, they gave him fruit. They put him in the bath twice a day, gave him a support to take pressure off his painful heel. They spigoted his catheter, emptied his bladder every two or three hours for a day or two, then tried him without the catheter, carefully showing him how to use a bottle, and ensuring that there was one where he could reach it on his left side. They sent for his clothes and shoes. They got him up, dressed, shaved, hair brushed, and showed him his image in the mirror. With the help of the physiotherapist they put him in a self-propelled wheel-chair and taught him how to use his good foot to drive himself about.

The physiotherapist mobilized his limbs and trunk, stood him up with support to give him the feel of the ground under his feet. The occupational therapist trained him to assist in his own dressing. The speech therapist discovered routes of communication by gesture and situational clues, and taught the relatives and the nurses how to exploit these. The doctor treated the accompanying urinary infection and anaemia, relieved pain, ensured sleep, conferred with relatives and with the therapeutic team. In the end the patient did not fully "recover" —but he regained self-respect and a limited degree of independence. He became much less demanding and frustrated. He was able to go on outings, and could spend an occasional weekend at home. He took up indoor gardening and filled the dayroom with pot plants. We did not "cure" him of his irremediable disease, but we were privileged to watch the tide of his personality begin to flow again over the dry sand of his disability.

PRINCIPLES

All this required the full geriatric team. In the more usual setting of the patient's home or a general hospital ward the same basic principles apply. These are:

(1) Listen carefully to the patient. He will tell you what needs to be done.

(2) Make yourself available to talk to relatives in privacy. They too have needs.

(3) Information is the fuel of opinion. So do not hesitate to investigate, but keep the investigation relevant to possible treatment.

(4) No form of treatment should be rejected dogmatically; always the benefits should be weighed against the hazards. To secure comfort in the last days of life risks are justified.

INVESTIGATION AND SURGICAL TREATMENT

The undiagnosed are often the unremedied; so no patient should be denied investigation. Evaluation of the haemoglobin, blood urea, electrolytes, and blood sugar is a minimum. A chest x-ray film may show unsuspected cancer, tuberculosis, or osteomalacia. Sternal marrow examination is well tolerated and should not be withheld on ground of age alone. Barium meals seldom lead to useful treatment. Barium enemas are more often helpful, but may be frustrated by non-retention or by faecal accumulations. Urine cultures often yield organisms, but their eradication less often relieves symptoms.

Surgery and anaesthesia are well tolerated, and should not be withheld if they offer hope of improvement in the quality of life. Post-operative rehabilitation may be very successful, and old people can learn to use colostomies or artificial limbs.

RELIEF OF SYMPTOMS

Intractable pain is mercifully rare in the elderly. Its adequate control requires timely relief with non-narcotizing doses of potent drugs, a technique which needs organization, but which yields benefits by relieving the fear of having to endure pain.

Dyspnoea is more common and more difficult to control. Good posture is best obtained at home by nursing the patient in a chair. Adequate diuresis is sometimes resisted, because the patient and his relatives become exhausted by frequent potting. A catheter should be used without hesitation. Oxygen usually causes more anxiety and tension than it relieves.

Anorexia is treated by indulgence. Favourite foods and beverages are prescribed; and a glass of whisky or sherry acquires a new and glorious flavour through having been prescribed by the doctor.

Treating dehydration is important, since ill old people do not experience thirst. Their fluid intake should be charted, aiming at an intake of 1,500 ml a day. If they have difficulty in swallowing they should use a straw or a child's feeding cup. Their fluids can be given in the form of jelly or liquidized foods.

Constipation is compounded by lack of roughage in the diet, lack of physical exercise, poor somatic muscle tone and evacuating power, inadequate opportunity, and fear of discomfort, quite apart from any autonomic dysfunction. The provision of a commode which the patient trusts and is prepared to use is as important as the prescription of the correct laxative or suppository. Regular enemas are required; regular rectal examinations are even more important.

Sleep disturbances send the doctor off on a prescription odyssey, sailing from drug to drug in an endeavour to secure sleep by night and wakefulness by day. From time to time one stops all drugs and starts again at the beginning with one aspirin at 9 p.m.—and sometimes this works. The hot milky drink may secure sleep at night, but the full bladder may alert early waking.

PSYCHOLOGICAL FEATURES

Doctors are often urged to allow old people to die with dignity. I find this very difficult to do, since I associate dignity with black silk hats, the measured tread, the grave nod of the head—at very least with ambulation, continence, and mental clarity—features which are lacking as death approaches. Near the end of life some old people become undignified, remove their clothing in public, and revile their dear ones with obscenities. Others lose self-control and become irritable, demanding, and selfish; refuse to be left alone; moan repetitively; ceaselessly ask for drinks; or demand to be taken to the lavatory, do nothing, then wet themselves. These anxiety symptoms are hard for relatives to bear; and many have confided to me that the last months of a loved parent's life were the worst they had ever experienced.

These situations test to the utmost the doctor's capacity to treat the irremediable. He must listen, sympathize, reassure, explain. The relatives require our ears and our time, but the doctor can also give practical help by arranging day hospital care or short-term admission.

CONCLUSION

Much of medical work is concentrated on the final months or year of life. The curative role of the doctor is being attenuated. But equal or greater professional satisfaction can be found by the skilled and perceptive treatment of "the irremediable."

Drug Therapy in the Elderly

BY

M. R. P. HALL

GENERAL PRINCIPLES

THE efficiency of the individual organs and the body lessens with age. For instance, renal function diminishes, enzyme induction is delayed, cell membrane composition and total body salt and water contents are altered, and lean body mass is reduced. Consequently, the elderly differ from younger people in their response to drugs, for their ability to handle drugs by absorption, detoxication, and excretion is naturally effected. Not surprisingly, therefore, iatrogenic disease related to drugs is very common.

Fortunately, as a rule, absorption is less affected by age than excretion and detoxication. Hence the failure of an elderly person to respond to an effective drug is nearly always due to failure of the patient to take the drug rather than to absorb it. Large loading doses of drugs are, therefore, rarely necessary and in most cases it is preferable to start with a small dose, particularly if the drug is potentially toxic and likely to be poorly excreted. This does not mean that large doses of some drugs should not be given to the elderly if indicated—for example, antibiotics in acute infections or diuretics in the early stages of heart failure. Nevertheless, in using drugs in the elderly it is wise to observe a few simple rules:

(1) Know the pharmacological action of the drug being used and in particular how it is metabolized and excreted.

(2) Use the lowest dose that is effective in the individual patient. Higher blood concentrations per dose are achieved and the half life of some drugs—for example, cortisol or digoxin—is prolonged in the elderly, and this can lead to accumulation and the need for lower and less frequent dosage. Drug dose should, therefore, be titrated with patient response.

(3) Use the fewest drugs the patient needs. Memory, particularly short-term memory, deteriorates with age; consequently complex drug regimens may be mismanaged.

(4) Do not use drugs to treat symptoms without first discovering the cause of the symptoms. These may sometimes be due to a social deprivation syndrome which may be better dealt with by a trained social worker.

(5) Do not withhold drugs on account of old age particularly when drug therapy may improve the old person's quality of life.

14

(6) Do not use a drug if the symptoms it causes are worse than those it is supposed to relieve. Hence knowledge of a drug's side effects is important and one should remember that sometimes adverse reactions may be individual to the patient and may occur to a drug which has been taken successfully for many years.

(7) Do not continue to use a drug if it is no longer necessary. It is a wise rule to review repeat prescriptions quarterly in all elderly patients.

DRUGS ACTING ON THE CARDIOVASCULAR SYSTEM

Heart failure is common in old age and digitalis glycosides remain the key to successful treatment. Their poor tolerance and adverse effects have been known for years. Possibly the use of the pure glycoside rather than a preparation of crude digitalis leaf and modern manufacturing techniques may have contributed to this intolerance. Ewy et al.[1] found that in the elderly the same dose of digoxin produced higher blood levels and longer blood half life. Rules (1) and (2) apply, and great care must be taken in the administration of all digitalis derivatives, the dose always being titrated against patient response. A dose of 0·25 mg daily is usually effective, though some individuals need less, in which case the small paediatric/geriatric (PG) tablets of 0·0625 mg strength may be useful. Maintenance therapy is probably unnecessary in about 70 % of cases[2] and the drug may be withdrawn in many instances quite safely.

That potassium depletion causes digitalis intolerance is well recognized. It may be produced not only by the use of powerful diuretics but may already exist as a result of reduced intake owing to poor diet. The serum potassium may be little guide to the total body potassium content, though low scrum levels are nearly always associated with low total body levels.[3]

Negative potassium balance in congestive heart failure may be high, and large potassium supplements are necessary when treating acute heart failure, particularly if diuretics are also used—for example, a minimum of 48 mEq/24 hr. Nevertheless, since impairment of renal function occurs with age, it may not be necessary for large doses to be given for long, and potassium levels should be closely monitored, the blood levels being checked at weekly intervals until the heart failure is controlled. Once heart failure is controlled, continued maintenance therapy with potassium salts may be unnecessary.[4] If potassium supplements are discontinued the patient must be watched for signs of hypokalaemia (confusion, lassitude, anorexia, cardiac arrhythmias, and muscular weakness) and blood levels checked at regular intervals, particularly if diuretics are continued.

Diuretics

Diuretics are commonly used in old people to treat heart failure and oedema. Indeed, they are probably over-used to treat dependent oedema, which is unlikely to respond, so that they produce sodium and potassium depletion, postural hypotension, immobility, constipation, faecal impaction with double incontinence, and a state of misery and social inacceptability. The actual drug used is a matter of personal choice, since most are effective—but probably bendrofluazide, chlorthalidone, and frusemide are the most useful. The dose should be large enough to be effective and very large doses—for example, frusemide 240 mg—may be necessary on occasions. It should be remembered that all diuretics may provoke gout and carbohydrate intolerance. Aldosterone antagonists such as spironolactone may potentiate their action and prevent excessive potassium depletion. Dall et al.[5] have reported that ameloride in combination with hydrochlorothiazide may conserve potassium. The drug, however, should be used with caution in the elderly since it may give rise to high blood potassium levels.

Beta-Blockers

The adrenergic β-receptor blockers may be used to control supraventricular arrhythmias in elderly patients. Practolol is probably the most useful since it is less likely to produce bradycardia, heart failure, and bronchospasm than propranolol. These drugs may be particularly useful in controlling the tachycardia associated with hyperthyroidism.

Hypotensive drugs should be used with caution in the elderly, and some physicians in geriatric medicine question their use at all. Nevertheless, rule (5) applies to this group of drugs and if their use enables the patient to lead a more pleasant and active life they should be used. The liability of some preparations to produce mental depression must be recognized.

The vasodilator drugs will increase peripheral circulation in the limbs as well as the cerebral circulation. Their use, therefore, to improve both the symptoms of peripheral vascular disease and the effects of cerebrovascular disease is advocated by their makers. Improvement in the efficiency of blood flow through diseased vessels, however, is doubtful and consequently their efficacy in improving symptoms. Nevertheless, some preparations do alter the metabolism of cells in the brain, so that some effect is a theoretical possibility. As a group of drugs they seem to produce little in the way of side effects even if their value remains unproved.

Drugs Acting on the Central Nervous System

The elderly commonly suffer from agitation, restlessness, and insomnia. In a busy clinic it is often difficult to elucidate the cause of these symptoms and hence drugs are frequently prescribed. Rule (4) particularly applies to these, for they are all potentially dangerous to the elderly. Nevertheless, they may be effective in relieving symptoms and hence useful. Some old people are extremely sensitive to some of these drugs: even quite small doses may produce soporific states, and hence small doses should be used initially.

Probably the most useful hypnotics are one of the modern chloral derivatives such as dichloralphenazone (Welldorm) or triclofos (Tricloryl). Alternatives to these are glutethimide (Doriden), which may give rise to cerebellar signs and vitamin D deficiency in some old people; chlormethiazole (Heminevrin); nitrazepam (Mogadon); and meprobamate (Miltown, Idemin, Equanil, Pathibamate, Mepavion). Barbiturates are not recommended, for the elderly tolerate them poorly and they may give rise to lethargy, depression, and confusion.

Sedatives and Tranquilizers

Of the sedatives and tranquilizers, the most widely used are diazepam (Valium) and chlordiazepoxide (Librium). Both drugs, however, may provoke a feeling of weakness in some old people—and patients who have had cerebrovascular accidents are particularly susceptible. Undoubtedly agitation and hallucinations are most easily controlled by the phenothiazine group. Despite its tendency to give rise to jaundice in some people, chlorpromazine (Largactil) is probably the most effective and widely used. Doses should be kept as small as possible. It is wise to start with a dose of 10 mg, increasing this as necessary. Alternatives are promazine (Sparine), which is weaker, and thioridazine (Melleril), which may be more effective in some patients. More potent drugs in this group are trifluoperazine (Stelazine) and haloperidol (Serenace); the latter, which comes in the form of colourless and tasteless drops, may be particularly useful in controlling the very agitated patient. The usual dose is 0·5 mg to 1·5 mg three times a day. Similarly the decanoate and enanthate forms of fluphenazine may be useful, since a single injection will control symptoms for quite long periods. It should be remembered that all these drugs produce side effects, and in particular features of Parkinsonism, so that it may be necessary to give an anti-Parkinsonian preparation simultaneously. They should also not be used in patients who are vulnerable to accidental hypothermia, and they may provoke postural hypotension.

The incidence of depressive illness rises with age and the treatment of patients with this condition should be supervised by a psychiatrist. Short courses of electro-shock therapy may often be more effective than long-continued drug taking. If drugs are used the tricyclic group of antidepressant drugs is most useful. These drugs may cause urinary retention, and constipation, and may precipitate or aggravate glaucoma. They may also provoke severe postural hypotension and aggravate dryness of the mouth—or even cause lingual or oral ulcers.

Rule (1) and (2) apply particularly to all these drugs but large doses should not be withheld from those patients who need them.

Parkinson's Disease

Treatment with L-dopa represents a considerable advance. It must, however, be used cautiously, for failure of treatment is often due to incorrect prescription. Thus the starting dose should not be greater than 125 mg daily, and increments should be at weekly intervals, and of 125 mg dose, until the daily dose equals 0·5 g. Some elderly respond to amantadine hydrochloride in an initial dose of 100 mg daily, which is increased to 100 mg twice daily after one week. Severe nausea and vomiting are common adverse reactions to L-dopa and may be due to peaking of blood levels, and a slow-release preparation prevents this. Consequently Brocadopa Temtabs may be the most appropriate L-dopa preparation for elderly patients. Optimum dosage may be lower than in younger people and improvement may continue for months or even years. The older anti-Parkinsonian drugs may have a place in the treatment of those patients who cannot tolerate L-dopa, but they should all be used with care, and rules (1) and (2) apply.

RELIEF OF PAIN

Pain and discomfort are common symptoms, being associated with skeletal disorders as well as with cancer.[6-8] Undoubtedly it is much easier to prevent the onset of pain than to relieve it once it has occurred. Pain should not be allowed to ebb and flow; hence analgesics, sedatives, anti-inflammatory drugs, and narcotics should be given regularly and patients instructed in their proper use to prevent the development of pain and minimize the symptom as much as possible.

Soluble aspirin probably remains the most effective and useful analgesic, particularly in the treatment of skeletal as opposed to visceral pain. The possibility of gastrointestinal bleeding must be remembered; some preparations—for example, benorylate, safapryn, or Caprin—may be safer but are more expensive. Paracetamol, either alone or in combination with other analgesics, is safer but less effective, though its absorption and consequently action may be enhanced by sorbitol. The anti-inflammatory drugs phenylbutazone (Butazolidin), oxyphenbutazone (Tanderil), indomethacin (Indocid), and ibuprofen (Brufen) are effective in relieving pain but all tend to give rise to gastrointestinal symptoms—though ibuprofen seems better tolerated by most of the elderly. Narcotics are often necessary to treat severe pain. If given in conjunction with chlorpromazine they may be used in quite small doses—for example, pethidine 150–300 mg daily—thus enabling the patient to remain alert yet be free from pain. In very severe pain diamorphine remains the drug of choice in combination with chlorpromazine.

Corticosteroids rarely need to be used and unless specifically indicated they should be avoided. They are sometimes useful for the treatment of arthralgia, which does not respond to other analgesics—for example, severe late-onset rheumatoid arthritis. Often prednisone, 1 or 2 mg three times a day, is effective. Similar doses may also be used in the treatment of asthma. Larger doses are necessary in the treatment of temporal arteritis and polymyalgia rheumatica. Here the initial dose should be high—reduction, which should be achieved as rapidly as possible, being titrated against the erythrocyte sedimentation rate. All patients on corticosteroids should also be given an anabolic steroid concomitantly in an attempt to prevent osteoporosis. Otherwise the regular use of anabolic steroids is probably of unproved value.

TREATMENT OF INFECTION

There are no special contraindications to the use of anti-bacterial drugs in the elderly. It should, however, be remembered that many are poorly eliminated; thus blood levels will be higher and toxic reactions may be more common. Antibiotic and antibacterial drugs should be given by mouth since injections may cause sterile abscesses and the resulting tissue breakdown may produce pressure sores. Concomitant monilial infections may occur in severely debilitated patients.

CONCLUSIONS

It is impossible in a short article such as this to cover all aspects of drug therapy in the elderly. For instance, replacement therapy using hormones such as thyroxine, or vitamins such as vitamin B_{12} and folic acid, may be necessary. Vitamins, particularly C and D, and minerals, such as iron, may be indicated in the housebound and other elderly prone to subnutrition. While there are no special preparations which will combat old age, the elderly will benefit as much from appropriate drug therapy as any young person. The key to good drug therapy is accurate diagnosis, assessment of the objectives of treatment, and use of the appropriate drug or drugs, bearing in mind the rules already outlined, which should govern the use of any drug. Good therapy is not easy but it is rewarding.

REFERENCES

1 Ewy, A., Kapadia, G., Yao, L., Lullin, M., and Marcus, F. I., *Circulation*, 1969, **39**, 449.
2 Dall, J. L. C., *British Medical Journal*, 1970, **2**, 706.
3 Cox, J. R., Pearson, R. E., and Speight, C. J., *Gerontologia Clinica*, 1972, **13**, 233.
4 Down, P. F., Polak, A., Rao, R., and Mead, J. A., *Lancet*, 1972, **2**, 721.
5 Dall, J. L. C., MacFarland, J. P. R., and Kennedy, R. D., *Proceedings of the VIth European Congress of Clinical Gerontology*, p. 371–373, 1971.
6 Sinclair, D., *British Journal of Hospital Medicine*, 1973, **9**, 568.
7 Merskey, H., *British Journal of Hospital Medicine*, 1973, **9**, 574.
8 Lipton, S., *British Journal of Hospital Medicine*, 1973, **9**, 583.

Cardiovascular Disease in the Old

BY

J. WEDGWOOD

In many cases cardiovascular disease in the old is similar to the disease in the young and middle aged, except that its pathology is weighted towards conditions such as ischaemic heart disease rather than congenital or rheumatic heart disease. This point, though perhaps obvious, needs to be made to emphasize that most forms of heart disease in the young which do not cause early death may be found in old age.

In other cases, particularly those presenting to the geriatric physician, and in patients over 75 or 80 years, the aetiology, symptoms, course and response to treatment are all considerably modified, and need separate consideration. The present paper is concerned with this group of patients and will deal with the commoner conditions in which the differences are most appreciable, and which present particular problems to the general practitioner. Congestive heart failure is a common condition covering most aspects of heart disease, and so this paper will be limited to a discussion of this condition.

The most outstanding feature of congestive heart failure is the ease with which elderly patients develop it and the relatively good response to treatment.[1] Congestive failure may develop in patients with less clinical evidence of heart disease than would be expected in younger patients. Though there is usually evidence of myocardial or valvular heart disease, precipitating factors are particularly important and need to be recognized before the condition can be adequately treated.

PRECIPITATING FACTORS

Chest Infection

Chest infection is a particularly important factor to bear in mind. Signs of bronchopneumonia may be difficult to detect, and relatively slight infection is often sufficient to precipitate failure. The combination of chest infection and heart failure in which it is difficult to decide the relative contribution of pulmonary and cardiac factors is common.

Atrial Fibrillation

Atrial fibrillation is common in the elderly, and may be paroxysmal. When the ventricular rate is rapid it is a common cause of failure. A more serious arrthymia is atrial flutter or atrial tachycardia with atrioventricular block. This condition is difficult to detect clinically except by

21

inspection of the venous pulse. When atrioventricular block is present with a 2 : 1 ventricular response the ventricular rate may be relatively slow and regular. It is particularly likely to occur in a patient who is being treated with digitalis for atrial fibrillation. It is a serious complication of digitalis toxicity, easily missed, and liable to be fatal.[2]

Heart Block

When the ventricular rate is slow, heart block may be a cause of congestive failure; this responds to measures which increase the ventricular rate. Stokes Adams attacks are the more dramatic effects of heart block, but congestive failure, chronic ill health, and confusional states may also be features of the slow ventricular rate. Artificial pacemaking is of value in these patients, and age should not prevent its use.

Cardiac Infarction

Silent cardiac infarction is common in the old or may present with

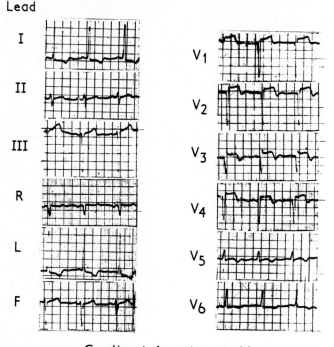

Cardiac infarction No. 66
F   89 years

FIG. 1—Acute anterior infarction in an 89-year-old woman without symptoms. (By kind permission of the publishers, Pitman Medical Publishing Co.Ltd. Wedgwood, J., in *Medicine in Old Age*, ed. J. Agate, p. 216. London, Royal College of Physicians, 1966.)

minor symptoms of confusion, weakness, or syncope, without chest pain (fig. 1).[3] It may also present with congestive failure and should be suspected in patients who develop failure without obvious cause. Clinical support for this diagnosis may be obtained from the sudden development of a gallop rhythm, which is often most easily heard over the lower sternum or xiphoid process in the old when auscultation is difficult.[4]

Subacute Bacterial Endocarditis

Between 20 and 30% of the cases of subacute bacterial endocarditis occur in patients over the age of 60.[5] The condition is easily missed in old age,[6] [7] but its insidious onset in the old may be associated with congestive failure and it should be suspected in patients with congestive failure, a heart murmur, and disproportionate constitutional symptoms; particularly if fever is present (fig.2).

Other Conditions

Other conditions which precipitate failure and may easily be missed are anaemia, thyrotoxicosis, myxoedema, and salt retention due to

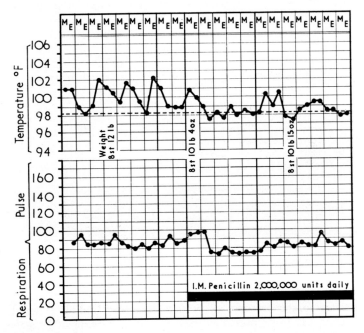

FIG. 2—Unexpected fever in a woman, aged 69, with subacute bacterial endocarditis.

treatment with steroids or with stilboestrol for carcinoma of the prostate. Pulmonary embolism is a fairly frequent cause of failure. Deep vein thrombosis is common and easily missed. Recurrent pulmonary embolism as a cause of failure may cause difficulty in diagnosis. Thiamine (aneurin, Vitamin B1) deficiency has been reported as a cause of congestive failure without the characteristic high output signs associated with beri-beri.[8] This condition does not appear to be common but may be being missed because it is not being suspected. Confirmation of thiamine deficiency may be obtained by estimating the red cell transketolase, but facilities for this are not often available. Treatment with thiamine is effective and may be diagnostic, but presents difficulties, [9] [10] so that its use as a diagnostic test is complicated.

UNDERLYING FACTORS

In most elderly patients myocardial disease is the underlying cause of failure. In about a quarter of the cases evidence of previous cardiac infarction or the presence of hypertension supports a diagnosis of ischaemic heart disease (table).[11] The remaining cases are usually considered to have ischaemic heart disease on rather less evidence. The precision of this diagnosis may be questioned but it remains a useful term and preferable to the obsolete "senile myocardial degeneration" which it replaced.

Heart Disease on Discharge or Death in Patients Aged 80 Years and Over

	M	F	Total	Total %
Ischaemic Heart Disease—Without Infarction	75	69	144	73
Ischaemic Heart Disease—With Infarction	19	20	39	20
Ischaemic Heart Disease—With Hypertension	0	6	6	3
Valvular Heart Disease	3	3	6	3
Cor Pulmonale	2	1	3	1
	99	99	198	100

(By kind permission of the publishers, Pitman Medical Publishing Co. Ltd. Wedgwood, J., in *Medicine in Old Age*, ed. J. Agate, p. 216. London, Royal College of Physicians, 1966.)

The post-mortem finding of brown atrophy of the myocardium is not related to the presence of failure. Necropsy finding of amyloid deposits in the heart muscle of elderly patients dying of congestive failure deserves more attention.[12] [13] This condition, known as senile cardiac amyloidosis, is at present a post-mortem diagnosis. Its incidence varies considerably in published series, but is particularly high in those over 90 years. It is associated clinically with extreme sensitivity to digitalis.

VALVULAR AND CONGENITAL HEART DISEASE, COR PULMONALE

Nearly all forms of congenital heart disease, except those associated with an early mortality, and of rheumatic and syphilitic heart disease have been found in old age (figs. 3 and 4).[14] Cor pulmonale occurs in elderly patients but is rare in the type of patient discussed here; though combinations of failure, chest infection, and emphysema, in which the aetiology is mixed, are common. Probably patients with congenital lesions or valvular heart disease acquired in earlier adult life who survive to these late ages do not develop failure until a myocardial factor is introduced.

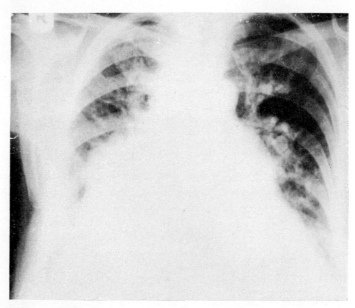

FIG. 3—Chest x-ray film. Woman aged 79 years with a ventricular septal defect. Confirmed at necropsy. (By kind permission of the publishers of the *Practitioner* and of Dr. K. M. MacKenzie. Wedgwood, J., *Practitioner*, 1968, 200, 778.)

Some forms of valvular heart disease, particularly mitral incompetence, may develop in old age as a result of cardiac infarction, ischaemic heart disease, calcification, or degenerative changes. Calcification of the mitral valve ring, calcium deposits near the ring, mucosal degeneration,[15] and changes in the chordae tendineae or

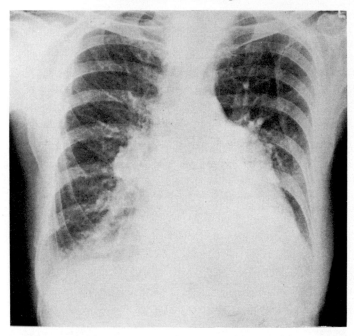

FIG. 4—Chest x-ray film. Woman aged 75 years with an atrial septal defect.

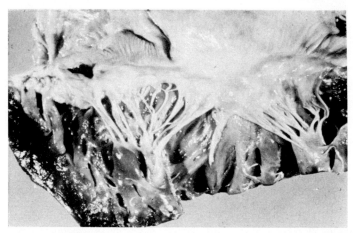

FIG. 5—Necropsy specimen showing degenerative changes in the mitral valve in a 90-year-old woman with mitral incompetence and intractable failure. (By courtesy of Dr. G. Farrer-Brown, Bland-Sutton Institute, Middlesex Hospital Medical School.)

papillary muscles may all cause mitral incompetence (fig. 5), which is sometimes severe and leads to intractable failure. Similar changes may occur in the aortic valve leading to mild stenosis or aortic incompetence from aortic ectasia.[14]

The difficulty of auscultation, and the fact that investigation is often not practicable or justified, means that our understanding of heart murmurs in these patients is inadequate. Systolic murmurs are difficult to assess, they may vary in length with the cardiac output, originate from more than one valve, or originate in an extracardiac arterial bruit in the abdomen or neck.

It is often difficult to estimate the haemodynamic significance of a suspected valvular lesion, but the importance of mitral incompetence of late onset as a cause of failure is easy to underestimate. The presence of a heart murmur should also be taken seriously because of the risk of bacterial endocarditis.

HYPERTENSION

Hypertensive heart disease is rare in the type of patient discussed here, though some degree of hypertension with ischaemic heart disease is common. The indication for using hypotensive drugs either for the relief of failure or on general principles is infrequent, and these drugs should hardly ever be used because of the risks of reducing the cerebral blood flow.

DIAGNOSIS

It is necessary to emphasize the importance of accurate diagnosis in congestive failure. The term is often used imprecisely to explain weakness, shortness of breath, or oedema of the ankles—for which there are many causes other than heart failure. Correct diagnosis is difficult but important since an incorrect diagnosis of heart failure may cause cardiac neurosis and greatly restrict the patient's rehabilitation and independence.

The diagnosis of congestive heart failure rests on careful examination of the venous pulse in the internal jugular vein. This is difficult in the old because of senile kyphosis and of the problem of positioning the patient. Arterial abnormalities in the neck may cause unusual pulsations or on the left side cause pressure effects which mimic a raised venous pressure.[16 17] Inspection should therefore be made of the right-hand side of the neck and, if there is difficulty in distinguishing an arterial from a venous pulse, pressure over the liver will elevate an abnormal venous pulse and over the lower part of the neck obliterate it.

Other signs of heart failure in the elderly tend to have equivocal significance. Rales at the lung bases can be found in many elderly patients who have been in bed.[18] The liver edge may be palpable owing to a low diaphragm or deformed rib cage. Oedema of the legs is common in the elderly without heart failure, though a sacral pad of oedema is perhaps more significant.

These difficulties emphasize the need for negative diagnosis. If the heart is not enlarged, there are no abnormal heart sounds, and the electrocardiogram is normal, heart failure is unlikely to be present. Palpation of the apex beat, auscultation, a chest x-ray film, and an electrocardiogram may be helpful in a negative way, though themselves may raise problems.

TREATMENT

The importance of precipitating factors in heart failure in the old has been mentioned and their recognition and treatment are of great importance. The diagnosis and treatment of concomitant chest infection with an appropriate antibiotic need particular emphasis. Signs in the chest may be minimal, and it is often justifiable to give an antibiotic on the suspicion that infection may be present if the response to treatment has otherwise been poor.

Diuretics

In the absence of atrial fibrillation, diuretics and the treatment of the precipitating cause are usually all that is needed. Digitalis should be kept in reserve unless atrial fibrillation is present. The choice and method of giving diuretics must take into account the problem of incontinence, and, in men, retention of urine if there is some prostatic obstruction. Elderly people may be weakened by the effort required to deal with a massive diuresis and do not stand up well to rapid changes in fluid and electrolyte balance. In most cases there is no need for the vigorous use of diuretics or for the more complex potent diuretics required in younger patients with severe or resistant failure.

The method and frequency of administration need thought. Elderly patients may not take tablets regularly or may spit them out after the nurse has left; in them the parenteral route may be better than the oral. After the acute phase is over diuretics may not need to be given daily. In maintenance therapy the diuretic can be given intermittently on the most convenient days. The patient should be regularly assessed and maintenance diuretics stopped as soon as possible. Diuretics tend to be continued after the problem of congestive failure has receded, from habit and because of difficulty in deciding that heart failure has ceased in the presence of factors such as leg oedema. If diuretics are given in small doses, intermittently, and for short periods, their complications such as potassium deficiency, gout, and (in the case of the thiazides) the provocation of diabetes, are less likely to occur and the patient's regimen is more easily managed.

Many of the above principles may seem obvious but are often neglected and more attention given to the nature of the diuretic itself. The *choice of diuretic* is of less importance except that the more potent and complex diuretic programmes are rarely needed. In the more serious or acute conditions frusemide has the advantage of powerful action, flexibility of dosage, and oral or parenteral administration. Given by mouth it acts within one hour and lasts for about eight hours. Its disadvantage is that it may be too effective—a problem that may be diminished by giving it in the smallest possible dose. In less serious states and for maintenance the thiazides are satisfactory. They act more slowly (within four hours) and last longer (for about twelve hours). Their prolonged action may be a handicap, as may their diabetogenic tendencies. Mersalyl is little used now but has advantages when a single injection is required, and it does not produce potassium deficiency. Moduretic (amiloride hydrochloride with hydrochlorothiazide) has recently been used in the elderly. It is said not to produce potassium deficiency.

Potassium Supplements

Potassium deficiency may be troublesome in the old and aggravate digitalis toxicity. Its occurrence is reduced if the general principles outlined are adhered to, but some form of potassium supplement is usually needed if the thiazides or frusemide are given. Such supplements do not obviate the need for regular assessment of patients on long-term diuretics. Though extra tablets are a nuisance for elderly patients, potassium supplements are more easily controlled if given separately. Slow K (Ciba) contains 600 mg of potassium chloride or 8 mEq of potassium. Two to six tablets a day may be given. Sando K (Sandoz) contains 12 mEq potassium as the chloride in effervescent tablets. The dose usually given is two to four tablets daily. The thiazide diuretics with slow release potassium offer the advantages of ease of administration but the disadvantage of a relatively small dose of potassium.

Digitalis

Digitalization is a considerable problem in elderly patients: thus digitalis intoxication is easily produced with small doses of the drug.[19] Mental confusion[20] is often the first indication of overdosage, or the patient may look or feel ill. Nausea and vomiting may occur later.

These symptoms are insidious and easily missed. The illness produced by digitalis in elderly patients has a most deleterious effect on their recovery, apart from the danger of atrial or ventricular arrthymias—which are common (fig. 6), more difficult to treat in the elderly than in the young, and often fatal. Digitalis needs to be given cautiously and the individual's response to it assessed by giving low doses in the first instance. Digoxin has the advantage of relatively quick action and excretion. Digoxin 0·25 mg three times a day is a large dose in old age, and 0·25 mg once or twice a day is often sufficient for the initial period. The maintenance dosage needs to be much smaller—0·125 mg or 0·0625 mg daily. Frequent observation of the patient is needed in

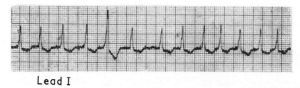

Lead I

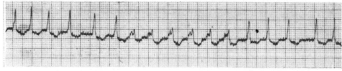

Lead I

FIG. 6—Ectopic arrthymia due to digitalis. E.C.G. Lead II. Woman aged 90 years. (By kind permission of the publishers of *Modern Medicine*.)

the early stages of treatment for early symptoms or signs, particularly arrthymias, of digitalis overdose. These should be taken seriously and the drug stopped at once if they occur. The danger of a large diuresis, or of potassium deficiency, aggravating the effects of digitalis should be borne in mind. Patients on long-term digitalis should be reviewed regularly and unless there is a good reason for continuing to give the drug it should be stopped.

The treatment of the elderly with digoxin has been further complicated by the discovery that the biological availability of the drug to the myocardium is influenced by the method of preparation.[21] [22] Different tablets of digoxin may have varying effects, though they contain the same amount of digoxin. At present the simplest solution to this problem is to digitalize and maintain each individual on the same brand of digoxin.

CONCLUSION

The symptomatology and course of cardiovascular disease is modified by age and there are several forms of heart disease specific to old age. Congestive failure is a common and often complex problem. With accurate diagnosis and careful treatment the prognosis is relatively good. The paradox of cardiovascular disease in the old is that, though heart disease is common in patients who survive to advanced old age, they are a selected group, a biological élite, whose general health and hearts might be expected to be unusually good.

I would like to thank Dr. G. Farrer-Brown, Senior Lecturer, Department of Pathology, The Middlesex Hospital Medical School for permission to publish Fig. 5, and Mr. G. Bryan, Chief Pharmacist, The Middlesex Hospital for his help and advice.

REFERENCES

[1] Bedford, P. D., and Caird, F. I., *Quarterly Journal of Medicine*, 1956, **25**, 407.
[2] Lown, B., and Levine, S. A., *Current Concepts in Digitalis Therapy*. London, Churchill, 1955.
[3] Pathy, M. S., *British Heart Journal*, 1967, **29**, 190.
[4] Evans, W. E., *British Heart Journal*, 1943, **5**, 205.
[5] Lerner, P. I., and Weinstein, L., *New England Journal of Medicine*, 1966, **274**, 199, 259, 388.
[6] Wedgwood, J., *Lancet*, 1955, **2**, 1058.
[7] Wedgwood, J., *Gerontologia Clinica*, 1961, **3**, Suppl., p. 11.
[8] McIntyre, N., and Stanley, N. N., *British Medical Journal*, 1971, **2**, 567.
[9] Pollitt, N. T., *Journal of the American Medical Association*, 1968, **203**, 153.
[10] Gould, J., *Proceedings of the Royal Society of Medicine*, 1954, **47**, 215.
[11] Wedgwood, J., in *Medicine in Old Age*, ed. J. Agate. London, Pitman Medical, 1966.
[12] McKeown, F., *Journal of Clinical Pathology*, 1963, **16**, 532.
[13] Pomerance, A., *British Heart Journal*, 1965, **27**, 711.
[14] Bedford, P. D., and Caird, F. I., *Valvular Disease of the Heart in Old Age*. London, Churchill, 1960.
[15] Pomerance, A., *British Heart Journal*, 1966, **28**, 815.
[16] Shirley-Smith, K., *British Heart Journal*, 1960, **22**, 110.
[17] Sleight, P., *British Heart Journal*, 1962, **24**, 726.
[18] Wood, P., *Diseases of the Heart and Circulation*, 2nd edn. London, Eyre and Spottiswoode, 1956.
[19] Wedgwood, J., *Modern Geriatrics*, 1970, **1**, 40.
[20] Durozier, P., *Gazette Hebdomadaire de Médecine et de Chirurgie*, 1874, **2**, 780.
[21] Hamer, J., and Chamberlain, D. A., *British Medical Journal*, 1973, **2**, 177.
[22] Falch, D., Teien, A., and Bjerkelund, C. J., *British Medical Journal*, 1973, **1**, 695.

Urinary Tract Diseases

BY

B. MOORE-SMITH

FOUR aspects of urinary tract diseases have been chosen for this article—uraemia, prostatic disease, urinary tract infection, and incontinence—and attention is drawn to some features of these conditions of particular importance in the elderly.

URAEMIA

The finding of a moderately raised blood urea (50–70 mg/100 ml) in elderly patients is so common as often to be regarded as normal—in the sense that it requires no immediate correction and is not accompanied by identifiable symptoms. Its presence, however, suggests an ageing kidney with progressive nephron depletion in the absence of other causes of a raised blood urea.

The other causes of uraemia may be divided into three parts—prerenal, renal and postrenal—but all these, of course, may be superimposed on existing nephron loss in an ageing kidney.

Prerenal Uraemia

Prerenal uraemia is due to inadequate glomerular filtration caused usually by such factors as haemorrhage, loss of extra-cellular fluid, or severely impaired cardiac output. In the elderly, minor states of dehydration are common, based on inadequate intake, and any further factor such as diarrhoea and vomiting or a silent myocardial infarction can produce an acute uraemic state, with confusion often as its leading symptom. The blood urea level may be as high as 200–250 mg/100 ml and will rapidly fall with adequate rehydration. A distinguishing feature in such cases is the maintenance of a normal or only moderately reduced plasma bicarbonate level.

Renal Uraemia

Any diffuse renal disease may be present in the elderly but probably the most common is chronic pyelonephritis. Diabetic nephropathy is less common, though diabetes is a common condition. The various forms of glomerulonephritis have their incidence chiefly earlier in life, and likewise hypertensive renal disease is relatively uncommon.

32

Postrenal Uraemia

The key to postrenal uraemia is obstruction to the flow of urine anywhere in the urinary passages. In both sexes chronic retention of urine based on faecal impaction is by no means uncommon and reinforces the necessity for routine rectal examination in the elderly. In men the commonest cause is prostatic enlargement and as many as 30% of men aged 80 and over have appreciable enlargement and often impaired flow. In women obstruction is less common but the presence of a cystocele may impair flow, and, particularly with complete procidentia, severe back pressure effects may result with the development of silent hydronephrosis. In these circumstances sudden death from acute renal failure over a matter of days may occur following a trivial alteration in renal perfusion.

MANAGEMENT

The management of acute renal failure by purely medical means is the same as in younger age groups and will not be discussed. The management of chronic uraemia depends primarily on the cause. The most immediately remediable causes, and also the commonest, lie in the prerenal group, and here the recognition of states of dehydration is important, while treatment with oral fluids is straightforward, provided it is adequately supervised. If there is any question of appreciable gastrointestinal tract loss appropriate replacement of electrolyte deficiencies is essential. A full assessment of the cardiovascular system, including an electrocardiogram, is necessary in any case of unexplained uraemia.

In postrenal causes of uraemia relief of the cause of the obstruction is the priority and age per se is no contraindication to surgery. The criterion for operation is the total clinical condition of the patient.

Provided underlying renal faction is preserved, relief of prerenal and postrenal factors will eliminate uraemia: in chronic renal failure, however, relief of the cause may well be impossible and treatment then becomes a matter of compensation for the renal defect so far as is possible. In the elderly renal dialysis or transplantation is unlikely to be justifiable, because of concomitant disease and disability as well as scarcity of resources.

In the management of chronic renal failure in the elderly it is especially important to ensure that the treatment is not worse than the disease and that the measures are simple and therefore more likely to be carried out. Some points to be observed include:

Fluid Intake

Urea excretion is proportional to urine flow and with low urinary output a slowly increasing "head" of urea and other metabolites builds

C

up in the plasma. This may be reduced by increasing the volume of urine passed and therefore the solute load excreted, even when the number of residual functioning nephrons is very severely reduced. In the elderly, however, the need to drink large quantities of fluid may be very difficult to communicate and resistance may be great, especially if there is a pre-existing degree of incontinence or lavatory facilities are inadequate. Even a moderate increase in urine flow is beneficial over a period of time. The help of relatives is invaluable in treating the patient outside hospital.

Ionic Balance

Sodium depletion may occur because of reduced sodium conservation and can cause further deterioration of renal function particularly during incidental illness. Potassium retention is well known with its dangers to the myocardium, and foods of high potassium content should be avoided as a general rule. A degree of acidosis is common and is usually well tolerated.

Protein

The elderly frequently eat a relatively high-carbohydrate, low-protein, diet and dietary control is not a major problem. Older people do not tolerate change and extreme dietary restrictions are not likely to be complied with.

Anaemia

Anaemia is invariable, is usually well tolerated, and is unresponsive to haematinics. Transfusion is only temporarily effective, hazardous, and best avoided.

Drugs

Elderly patients are frequently more sensitive to drugs of all types and in chronic renal failure drugs partly or entirely excreted through the kidneys may quickly reach toxic serum levels. This is especially true of antibiotics, and tetracyline in particular may raise the blood urea level even further. Conversely urinary tract infection may be more difficult to treat because of lack of excretion and this is especially true of nitrofurantoin and nalidixic acid.

PROSTATIC DISEASE

The usual presentation of prostatic disease—increasing difficulty in micturition—may be masked in the elderly, and the initial symptoms may be haematuria, or, as with younger patients, acute retention precipitated by diuretic therapy or anticholinergic drugs. Less widely recognized perhaps are dribbling incontinence due to retention with overflow and unrecognized acute retention causing a confusional state. A uraemic syndrome in a man always requires exclusion of prostatic obstruction as a cause. Treatment at present is essentially surgical and good results in suitable patients at any age are to be expected. Trials of various hormone preparations hold hope for future medical management.

Carcinoma of the prostrate is the commonest neoplastic disease of the elderly man, said to be present in 95% of histologically examined prostates in the 8th decade. Presentation may be through urinary symptoms but not uncommonly is due to metastatic disease. In particular the diagnosis should be thought of in previously fit men in their 80's and 90's who complain of nothing more than mild malaise or whose social behaviour deteriorates for no apparent reason over a short time. Bone pain, particularly in the lumbosacral spine or pelvis, is a relatively frequent metastatic presentation but very widespread bony metastases may be asymptomatic. The plasma acid phosphatase level is variable but is frequently raised, sometimes to very high levels, and with extensive bone involvement a raised alkaline phosphatase and sometimes a peripheral blood picture of leucoerythroblastic anaemia may be seen. Treatment with oestrogens in most instances is successful and lengthy remissions are frequently seen.

URINARY TRACT INFECTION

The spontaneous rate of urinary tract infection in women seen in domiciliary practice is said to be around 2%, but surveys in the elderly have found rates of around 20% in Britain, and in hospital rates as high as 67% have been quoted; in men spontaneous infection below the age of 70 is rare but its occurrence is said to be similar to that in women above this age. Possibly a prostatic antibacterial factor may account for this difference between the sexes at younger ages.

In elderly men collection of a reliable mid-stream urine specimen (MSU) is relatively straightforward; in elderly women, on the other hand, it is a task of some difficulty and the average MSU is almost certainly not midstream, and infrequently composed solely of urine. Thus urine specimens from elderly women submitted for bacteriological examination are often contaminated from various sources and this is reflected in the reported results of culture, before which the specimen may frequently be "incubated" at room temperature for several hours. This last difficulty is obviated by "dip slide" techniques, but the reliability of the results of a specimen "dipped" still remains in some doubt. In hospital conditions MSUs in elderly women have been shown to have a 57% false-positive rate, and though suprapubic aspiration gives totally reliable specimens, it is technically unsuitable for routine use. Alexa bag specimens show a similar order of reliability and could be used to check "abnormal" MSUs.

The interpretation of the results of laboratory examination depends primarily on the quantitative bacterial count. Significant infection is associated only with bacterial counts above 100,000/mm^3. There must be only one organism and in domiciliary practice this is likely to be *Escherichia coli* or a proteus in a pure culture. Two or more organisms reported as co-existing are due to contamination no matter how high the count. The presence or absence of pus cells is in general unhelpful and microscopical haematuria is uncommon.

Infection of the upper urinary tract in elderly patients is very difficult to establish. The classical clinical picture of acute pyelonephritis is uncommon and chronic pyelonephritis, though common (6% in one survey) as a post-mortem finding, is seldom accompanied by local symptoms in life. Suspicion may be aroused by heavy pyuria, or the results of a plain x-ray film or pyelography.

Treatment

Significant bacteriuria is likely to be asymptomatic in the elderly even more than in the younger age groups. It should be treated because of the deleterious effects of urinary infection on renal function, which is already likely to be compromised, as well as the known high incidence of chronic pyelonephritis. Fluids should be greatly encouraged, any fear of dilution of antiboitic concentration being far outweighed by the decreased reproduction rate of *E. coli* in diluted urine and the washout effect of the high urine flow on the bacterial numbers. The vast majority of *E. coli* found in domiciliary practice will be sensitive to sulphonamides, which are safe and effective. Otherwise, antibiotic treatment should follow the sensitivities found on culture and with appropriate manipulation of the urinary pH to match the organism concerned and the antibiotic chosen.

The length of treatment for a straightforward urinary infection is customarily one week and for acute pyelonephritis two weeks. In chronic pyelonephritis recommendations for length of treatment vary from six weeks to six months, using rotating antibiotics, but there is little further evidence as to their efficacy or necessity. A short (two-week) initial course with careful follow-up is probably preferable.

Relapse or re-infection is as common as in the younger age groups; if it persists, investigation is required to determine the cause, as treatment will be without lasting benefit until the cause is eliminated. By the same token a urinary infection should always be checked after treatment to confirm relief and, if pyelonephritis is suspected, at monthly intervals for at least six months.

INCONTINENCE

When the intravesical pressure exceeds the urethral resistance voiding normally occurs; voiding becomes incontinence when it happens in an uncontrolled fashion. In the elderly lack of adequate higher cerebral control is often an important cause, though the local mechanisms remain intact. This is seen transiently in early strokes, acute confusional episodes and states of altered consciousness, and epilepsy. It may also be seen in some frontal lobe lesions and particularly in established dementia.

Despite normal higher cerebral control, environmental factors may be vitally important as a source of apparent incontinence when access to the lavatory is restricted or it is too far away, or toilet rounds are inflexible, or attendants fail to realize that the matter is urgent. Being bed- or chair-fast are powerful overriding factors. Rarely with normal higher control and intact bladder mechanisms psychological factors may underlie apparent incontinence as a facet of a "call for help".

Local causes affecting the bladder mechanisms may firstly over-stimulate the detrusor by irritating it, as in acute cystitis, bladder stone, or neoplasm. All these cause urgency, and incontinence if help is not at hand. How far urinary infection on its own is responsible for incontinence is less certain. After many months of contracting against prostatic obstruction the detrusor may dilate, become unable to expel the last part of the urine, and finally become an inert and grossly distended bag stretching the bladder neck and causing continuous dribbling incontinence. Stress incontinence in women is fairly common in the elderly and depends on the altered anatomical relationship between the bladder neck and urethra, on the one hand, and the pelvic floor, on the other. Urethral resistance is sometimes diminished by invasion by prostatic carcinoma resulting in dribbling incontinence; otherwise urethral malfunction is almost unknown as a cause of incontinence.

Interference with the nerve supply to the bladder will also interfere with the balance between the detrusor and the urethra plus the external sphincter. Thus incontinence may result from a wide variety of causes, from cord lesions to peripheral neuropathy. In multiple sclerosis, for instance, there is frequently a progession from detrusor over-activity early, with incontinence, to increased outflow resistance later, with retention.

Treatment

Local causes require local treatment and must always be sought before accepting incontinence as being due to loss of higher control. The transient causes may be allowed to resolve as the underlying condition improves, while environmental factors in particular should be amenable to alteration and explanation. The importance of getting the patient out of bed with its connotations of helpless dependence cannot be overemphasized. Also of vital importance is the avoidance of unnecessary hypnotics and the initiation of regular toiletting and habit training, which can often greatly improve incontinence of so-called cerebral origin. Surgical help should always be sought in appropriate circumstances.

In some instances, despite correction of all remediable abnormalities, the patient is left with intractable incontinence. In women, especially if confused, it is impossible to fit an adequate external appliance, though some devices are suitable for the mentally alert and well motivated. A catheter is therefore the only practical solution and if of small size, with a small bag and adequately cared for, success for a period of years can be obtained and infection is rarely a major problem. In men long-term catheterization can cause troublesome periurethral problems, but in practice the relief to all concerned outweighs these dangers and a successful catheter life can be led for many months or even years. Before inserting a catheter, however, consideration should be given to the wide variety of incontinence appliances available. If fitted carefully these may be of considerable help, especially when the patient is out of bed. Nearly all appliances suffer from reflux problems in bed and considerable co-operation by the patient is needed for success. Electronic implants for increasing outflow resistance may help in selected cases of both sexes and are under continuing development.

FURTHER READING

Agate, J. N., *The Practice of Geriatrics*, 2nd ed. London, William Heinemann Medical Books, 1970.
Brocklehurst, J. C., Dillane, J. B., Griffiths, L., and Fry, J., *Gerontologia Clinica*, 1968, **10**, 242.
Brumfitt, W., and Reeves, D. S., *Journal of Infectious Diseases*, 1969, **102**, 61.
Jones, N. F., and Wing, A. J., in *International Handbook of Medical Science*, 2nd ed., ed. by D. Horrobin and A. Gunn. Oxford, Medical & Technical Publishing Co., 1972.
Kass, E. H., *Transactions of the Association of American Physicians*, 1956, **69**, 56.
Lancet, 1968, **1**, 732.
Lancet, 1968, **1**, 1183.
McMillan, J., and Linton, A. L., *Gerontologia Clinica*, 1968, **10**, 58.
Moore-Smith, B., *Modern Geriatrics*, 1971, **1**, 124.
Shuttleworth, K. E. D., *British Medical Journal*, 1970, **4**, 727.
Stamey, T. A., Fair, W. R., Timothy, M. M., and Chung, H. K., *Nature*, 1968, **218**, 444.
Stamey, T. A., Pfau, A., *California Medicine*, 1970, **113**, 16.
Wing, A. J., *British Medical Journal*, 1970, **3**, 753.
Wing, A. J., *British Medical Journal*, 1970, **4**, 35.
Woodford-Williams, E., *British Journal of Clinical Practice*, 1960, **14**, 351.

Care of the Elderly in General Practice

BY

CHARLES HODES

By mid 1971 the population of the retirement ages—65 years and over, men and women—had increased by 15% since 1961. By 1981 this population will have risen again by a similar amount.[1] The average list size per general practitioner is now about 2,500 and therefore he provides general medical services for 300 patients over 65 years of age, with about 100 of these being over 75. The development of the health team[2] in recent years has enabled the general practitioner to approach the care of the elderly more from the point of view of prevention and early diagnosis,[3][4] and new developments with social workers in general practice[5] may bring further benefits.

The assessment of the patient's needs and the organization of the care required are the essential tasks of the general practitioner. These needs may be known or unknown to the patient. At least six different aspects should be considered.

THE PRIMARY CARE TEAM

The general practitioner, the health visitor, and the district nurse together can provide the best care for the elderly in their own homes. Working from a common centre and sharing one medical record, there is adequate opportunity for exchange of information—which is so important in giving personal medical care to patients who often have some degree of mental confusion, in addition to the usual spectrum of diseases. Age is not a barrier to attendance at the surgery, and in fact the elderly patient should be encouraged to remain mobile and attend as required. Consultation with the health visitor and treatment by the district nurse should also be available at the surgery. Appointments —making and keeping—are easily overlooked by the elderly and it helps if they are always given an appointment in writing and a sympathetic receptionist fits them in without too much waiting if an appointment has not been made. Though willing relatives and friends may help increasingly with their own cars, more organized transport services[6] in general practice are required if the preventive approach is to increase.

Information about the services available locally should be kept at every practice. Local authorities often have booklets of services and can provide well-illustrated pamphlets on such subjects as diet and exercise; the health visitor is of course the best person to give out this information and can supplement it with individual consultation and with patient groups. Group discussions are also helpful in preparing for retirement,[7] and health education in the elderly should also be concerned with the prevention of accidents and fire safety. Local clubs, laundry services, washing facilities, chiropody, and meals-on-wheels are generally available and should be introduced to patients even if only required occasionally. Convalescent holidays are especially worthwhile in the elderly and whenever possible should include both husband and wife.

Nurses' Role

The nurse has been identified more with the care of the elderly sick patient. She can be supported in her work in the home by bath attendants and male nurses, who are playing an increasingly important part in the care of the male geriatric patient. Night nursing may also be available and if required only for a short time can make hospital admission unnecessary. Visits to the home for routine injections can be used as a method of surveillance and any change be reported to other members of the team.

At present there is little in the way of domiciliary physiotherapy but the district nurse can give help with breathing exercises for the chest infection and continuing support for the patient with a hemiplegia. Aids to nursing—such as commodes, bed rests, and disposable bedding supplies—are always available. Laboratory services are now used extensively by general practitioners, and the district nurse can take urine and blood specimens in the home and return them to the surgery for collection by the hospital transport services. For haemoglobin estimation a Spence Haemoglobinometer is very simple and quick to use, in both the home and surgery, and when any anaemia is due to poor diet the health visitor can soon call at home with advice and help.

Practice Premises

Practice premises have changed considerably in recent years and very large centres may present problems for the older patient. Cars should be able to drive up to the front entrance of the building, the doors should be wide enough for a wheelchair, and preferably there should be no steps. When all the members of the team have their own accommodation in the building referral is simpler and joint consultation can deal with problems quickly. A sufficient number of warm examination rooms allow the patients to dress and undress at their usual speed, and they can be helped by a receptionist or nurse; this also permits the general practitioner to carry on with other duties.

Good communication is facilitated by regular meetings between members of the primary care team. A high standard of record keeping is important and the problem-orientated record[8] may be found useful in geriatric care. All patients should keep with them at all times a treatment card, which can be used for repeat prescriptions and give useful information to any doctor seeing the patient as an emergency without the medical record being available.

Studies on the unreported needs of old people[9] and an evaluation of early diagnostic services for the elderly[10] have indicated the need for preventive care. To carry this out in general practice requires an age-sex register from which the geriatric register can be constructed.[11] [12] Invitations for examinations can be sent to selected patients, and these screening examinations can be carried out by the primary care team in the surgery and in the home; treatment and follow-up are carried out as required. Special registers for high-risk groups, such as patients living alone and the surviving partner on the death of a spouse, are indicated.

SOCIAL SERVICES

The elderly patient depends on the social services as well as the primary medical care team to live in the community. The social worker's client and the general practitioner's patient are the same person, and working together can only improve the total care of the elderly. If the social worker can use the general practitioner's premises, regular communication is more likely and the preventive approach possible. They many benefits now available in the way of financial help and housing are best dealt with by the social worker. Psychogeriatric cases need the support of the social work services and patients recently discharged from hospital can be followed by a worker who is in close contact with the psychiatric services. The home help, in addition to cleaning and shopping duties, is a great support for the often depressed and isolated patient, and can alert the general practitioner if there is any deterioration.

When the elderly patient can no longer manage at home, the social worker will arrange alternative accommodation. This may be in a flat or bungalow with a supervising warden. If this is not sufficient, residential accommodation can be provided on a temporary or permanent basis. The temporary care may be used when a relative has to go into hospital or goes off on holiday; it may also be used for day care when meals are provided and occupational therapy is available. This also relieves the isolation of the permanent residents, bring them into contact with their community, and introduces the temporary residents to what might become their home.

By arrangement with the local authority, the general practitioner may provide medical care for the residents. In this work he can be supported by the health visitor and district nurse. It is useful to have an assessment chart for patients in addition to the usual medical records, which can be shared by the primary medical care team. The chart is used to record essential information about the patients, and to note changes which occur with time. The first part can be completed by the health visitor, and gives a score based on assessments of physical state, mental state, activity, mobility, and incontinence. If the score rises, the patient is deteriorating. The second part is completed by the nurse on admission and then periodically as indicated; there is a scoring system for hearing and the state of the feet.

MEDICAL SERVICES

The geriatrician and his social worker in the local hospital are now very much part of community care and should be well known by the general practitioner. Domiciliary visits should be readily available without undue delay and requested for assessment and opinion, not only for admission. This prevents crisis from developing and allows the geriatrician to plan his admissions. The increase in the number of psychogeriatric patients in general practice gives rise to problems of regular medication and also to over-dosage; close supervision is required of patients living alone. The inclusion of geriatric and psychiatric services in new district hospitals will strengthen the support given to general practitioners.

Refractive errors are common and old spectacles may have been worn for may years; simple tests for visual acuity can be done in general practice but the detection of glaucoma requires special equipment and should be carried out by an ophthalmologist. During school holidays a technician with suitable equipment may be "borrowed" from the local authority for sight testing in old people's homes. Hearing aids are usually given out by special centres and often involve further travel for examination and fitting; patients of any age may benefit by an aid and there should be regular supervision of its use and performance.

THE COMMUNITY

The elderly patient usually wishes to continue to be independent and is supported by family and neighbours. The general practitioner can help by providing and introducing skilled help. The voluntary societies such as the British Red Cross and WRVS and help given by local groups such as Rotary are most valuable. Group practices and health centres can have groups of "friends," who give help of all kinds to the elderly.

THE PATIENT

Old people often do not come forward for care—medical and social. This reluctance may be less in relation to the family doctor who is a familiar face, and the health visitor and nurse working with him are identified by the patient as part of the same care. An understanding of the patient's attitude is therefore important, and a health education programme can be introduced which promotes early diagnosis and the acceptability of any treatment offered. When an elderly patient is dying at home the primary care team needs all its skills. They can offer complete care when the patient may need them most and can continue to support the bereaved.

THE FUTURE

The identification of the elderly in general practice is essential for a preventive programme, and it is to be hoped that executive councils will provide geriatric age-sex registers as a regular service. They may, of course, come within the province of the district community physician in 1974, and perhaps he will also supply the transport for patients which will facilitate better care. Easier communication by provision of more telephones is needed. The provision of more day centres and day hospitals will enable the care of the elderly in general practice to continue at a high standard.

REFERENCES

[1] Department of Health and Social Security, On the State of the Public Health. London, H.M.S.O., 1971.
[2] Royal College of General Practitioners, Present State and Future Needs of General Practice. 3rd edn. London, Royal College of General Practitioners, 1973.
[3] Hodes, C., Journal of the Royal College of General Practitioners, 1971, 31, 469.
[4] Williams, E. I., et al., British Medical Journal, 1972, 3, 445.
[5] Goldberg, E. M., and Neill, J. E., Social Work in General Practice. London, Allen and Unwin, 1972.
[6] Lance, H., Journal of the Royal College of General Practitioners, 1971, 21, Suppl. No. 3.
[7] Harte, J. D., Journal of the Royal College of General Practitioners, 1972, 22, 612.
[8] Weed, L. L., Medical Records, Medical Education and Patient Care. Cleveland, Ohio, 1971.
[9] Williamson, J. et al., Lancet, 1964, 1, 1117.
[10] Lowther, C. P., MacLeod, R. D. M., and Williamson, J., British Medical Journal, 1970, 3, 275.
[11] Hodes, C., Journal of the Royal College of General Practitioners, 1968, 15, 286.
[12] Forbes, J. A., British Medical Journal, 1969, 2, 46.

Non-Specific Presentation of Illness

BY

H. M. HODKINSON

PRESENTATION of illness in the elderly is often misleadingly different from that in younger age groups, and in particular, it may be entirely non-specific. Some differences may reflect the altered responses of the elderly in mechanisms such as the production of fever or pain. For example, myocardial infarction occurs quite commonly in the elderly but is usually not accompanied by typical transverse chest pain and shock. Often pain is totally absent and the patient presents with an episode of collapse, confusion, or breathlessness. Similarly in the old, lobar pneumonia—instead of having its presence indicated by cough, fever, and leucocytosis, as in the young—may present insidiously with confusion, drowsiness, unsteadiness, and slight breathlessness. These vague patterns of illness are common in the elderly and this article will consider some of the more frequent presenting syndromes.

"FAILURE TO THRIVE"

Illness quite often presents as an insidious and progressive physical deterioration, for which the paediatric term "failure to thrive" is appropriate. Typically the patient's decline comprises deteriorating social competence, weight loss, loss of appetite, increasing frailty, and diminishing initiative, concentration, and drive. This general failure of the old person is all too often accepted as due to "old age" or senility or is regarded as a dementing process and the physical basis is overlooked. There are many diagnostic possibilities.

Malignant Disease

Malignant disease in the old quite often presents in this way. The common primary sites are lung, breast, prostate, colon, and rectum. A chest x-ray film and rectal examination, and examination of the breasts in women, are therefore essential parts of the assessment of the elderly patient with an unexplained general deterioration. Diagnosis may lead to useful therapy: stilboestrol treatment is often helpful in cancer of the breast or prostate even when there is wide metastasis while resection may be advisable for colorectal growths.

Endocrine and Metabolic Disorders

Endocrine and metabolic disorders also need to be considered. Thyroid disease is particularly difficult to recognize clinically in the old.

Perhaps half the patients with hypothyroidism do not show a classical myxoedematous picture but present with apathy, depression, mental, and physical slowing or entirely non-specific deterioration.[1] Hyperthyroidism rarely presents a classical clinical picture in the elderly and has a fairly high incidence in ill old people.[1] It may present as "apathetic thyrotoxicosis,"[2] with physical lethargy and mental depression or with general debility, perhaps accompanied by cardiac failure and sometimes auricular fibrillation but with none of the other usual stigmata of thyrotoxicosis. In view of the fairly high prevalence, difficulty of clinical recognition, and the treatable nature of thyroid disease, there is a strong case for performing thyroid function tests routinely in ill old people. On the other hand, a single result of estimating the protein-bound iodine, T-3 uptake, or T-4 level may be misleading because of the common occurrence of reduced thyroxine-binding globulin in ill old people, so that both the protein-bound iodine level (or T-4) and T-3 uptake need to be determined.[3]

Diabetes is another common disease and may also produce failure to thrive rather than present classically. It is easily missed, as glycosuria may not occur owing to high renal threshold; a random blood sugar measurement is a far more reliable screening test.[4] Uraemia is a further diagnostic possibility and is most often due to chronic pyelonephritis.

In old people who fail to thrive there is thus considerable value in doing laboratory screening tests, and these would most usefully include: measurements of the levels of blood urea, electrolytes, glucose, haemoglobin, T-3, and protein-bound iodine or T-4.

CNS Diseases

Diseases of the central nervous system may also present unobtrusively. Parkinsonism is often overlooked, being common in old age but missed because tremor is either absent or slight and the typical rigidity may not be noticed. Doctors need to look actively for the disease as L-dopa therapy can so often make a worthwhile contribution. Multiple minor strokes and the development of a pseudobulbar syndrome are less likely to be overlooked but ignoring peripheral neuropathy is an occasional pitfall; malignant disease or diabetes is the commonest cause of this condition.

Depression

Depression is another possibility that is very commonly overlooked, both in general practice and in hospital. Depression is common in old age but may often present an atypical picture, masquerading as physical disease or as failure to thrive. The possibility of depression must always be kept in mind by doctors dealing with the elderly. Inquiry about the cardinal symptoms of depression—early waking and anorexia—may often reveal the diagnosis, further questioning of the seemingly cheerful old person uncovering gross depressive or suicidal ideas. Treatment of depression in the old is usually with one of the tricyclic antidepressants and the results are often gratifying.

Chronic Infections

Chronic infections are a somewhat unusual cause of insidious decline but, though uncommon, pulmonary tuberculosis—particularly in the elderly man—and subacute bacterial endocarditis must be remembered as possibilities because of their seriousness and treatment potentiality.

Iatrogenic Illness

Iatrogenic illness should always be considered. The elderly are particularly vulnerable to the adverse effects of drugs,[5] and examples in the context of failure to thrive include over-sedation from night sedatives (especially barbiturates), anti-epileptic drugs or tranquillizers depression from reserpine-containing drugs, drug-induced Parkinsonism from phenothiazines, and weakness due to hypokalaemia following diuretic therapy with inadequate potassium supplementation.

FALLS AND BLACKOUTS

This is another important presentation of illness in the elderly and because of accompanying trauma or fracture often leads to hospital admission. Patients with Parkinsonism are particularly prone to repeated falls, while those with unstable knees from osteoarthritis are also particularly vulnerable. Patients with rheumatoid arthritis affecting the cervical spine may have falls owing to vertebrobasilar insufficiency which occurs on moving the neck. So-called "premonitory falls" may herald acute physical illness such as pneumonia.

The side effects of drugs also need to be considered in the list of causes. Hypotensive drugs are commonly to blame for falls and blackouts, and all too often these have been prescribed on flimsy grounds, the patient not having true sustained hypertension. Here the mechanism is that of postural hypotension and this may also result from over-enthusiastic diuretic therapy that has lowered the serum sodium level. Over-sedation with barbiturates or phenothiazine tranquillizers may also result in falls.

MENTAL DETERIORATION

Very commonly, physical illness may present as mental disturbance in the elderly patient, and it is important that such mental symptoms are not mistakenly ascribed to dementia or "senility". The possibility of a physical cause for mental symptoms most obviously needs to be considered when these are of recent onset.

Acute Confusional States

These may be due to wide variety of diseases,[6] but most important among these are lobar pneumonia, bronchopneumonia, urinary infection, cardiac failure, and left ventricular failure. Though confusional states may readily occur in patients whose previous mental state was completely normal, pre-existing dementia and Parkinsonism both appear to facilitate their development.[6] Drug therapy may also result in confusional states. Barbiturates, tricyclic antidepressants, and anti-Parkinsonian drugs are specially noteworthy. Among the anti-Parkinsonian drugs, the atropine-like drugs such as benzhexol and orphenadrine are often implicated, but amantidine may give confusional states remarkable for the intensive visual hallucinations which may accompany them.

Subacute and chronic confusional states are particularly likely to be confused with dementia and here such causes as uraemia, carcinomatosis, pernicious anaemia, or hypothyroidism need to be considered.

Organic brain disease may also result in true dementia. In some instances an accurate diagnosis—for example, that of cerebral arteriosclerosis or a cerebral tumour—may not lead to any therapeutic opportunities, but the diagnosis of rarer diseases such as subdural haematoma, low pressure hydrocephalus,[7] or general paresis is important as these are potentially reversible.

"Rheumatism"

Poorly localized skeletal or muscular aches and pains are so common in old age because of the high incidence of degenerative joint disease that "rheumatic" pains heralding treatable or serious disease may unwisely be ignored. Osteomalacia is an important example as it is far from rare, eminently treatable, but easily overlooked. It affects particularly the housebound, those with previous gastric surgery, and women as opposed to men.[8] The patient becomes progressively more disabled, with "rheumatic" pains and proximal muscle weakness as the key symptoms. They may develop a typical waddling "penguin" gait and have special difficulty in getting up from a chair because of the muscle weakness.

Another important cause of "rheumatic" pain is the presence of metastases in bone. These occur mostly commonly from carcinoma of breast or prostate and may respond well for a time to treatment with stilboestrol. Multiple myeloma deposits are another possibility. The recent development of low back pain in an elderly person is not rarely due to these conditions, whereas prolapse of the intervertebral disc is practically never the explanation and simple osteoporotic collapse uncommonly so.

IMMOBILITY

An old person "going off his feet" is a common reason for admission to a geriatric department. Again, all too frequently this is assumed to be simply due to old age and the physical basis overlooked. Central nervous system disease—especially strokes or Parkinsonism—and locomotor disease such as osteoarthritis, rheumatoid arthritis, or osteomalacia are major causes. It is not rare for fracture to have been missed as the cause for immobility in patients who have had many falls. Immobility may also develop because of general frailty in the context of failure to thrive or may be due to loss of confidence due to frequent falls or unsteadiness—for example, from laterally unstable knees in severe osteoarthritis, postural hypotension, or over-sedation.

INCONTINENCE

Incontinence too should not automatically be accepted as due to old age or mental deterioration. Immobility itself may cause incontinence and other major factors are urinary infection; urinary retention with overflow; stress incontinence in old women who have had children; faecal impaction giving either urinary retention or spurious diarrhoea and faecal incontinence; and incontinence associated with the urgency caused by diuretic therapy. Night sedation may be responsible for incontinence during the night.

CONCLUSION

All these examples show that presentation is often misleading or obscure in elderly patients—a factor which calls for special vigilance in dealing with the elderly. Unless full use is made of good history taking (particularly with regard to drug therapy) physical examination, and relevant investigations, many errors will be made. The non-specific presentation of illness in the old must be regarded as a diagnostic challenge. If this attitude is adopted, medical work with the elderly becomes a fascinating, exacting, and rewarding discipline. Only by proper diagnosis can the elderly be helped to the full. If their symptoms are dismissed and "old age", "senility", "rheumatism", or some other conveniently vague label is applied, many opportunities for effective treatment of old patients will be missed, at the cost of much unnecessary suffering and disability.

REFERENCES

[1] Jefferys, P. M., *Age and Ageing*, 1972, **1**, 33.
[2] *Lancet*, 1970, **2**, 809.
[3] Jefferys, P. M., Farran, H. E. A., Hoffenberg, R., Fraser, P. M., Hodkinson, H. M., *Lancet*, 1972, **1**, 924.

[4] Denham, M. J., *Age and Ageing*, 1972, **1**, 55.
[5] Wade, O. L., *Age and Ageing*, 1972, **1**, 65.
[6] Hodkinson, H. M., *Journal of the Royal College of Physicians*, 1973, **7**, 307.
[7] *British Medical Journal*, 1973, **2**, 260.
[8] Conacher, W. D. H., *Practitioner*, 1973, **210**, 351.

Diet in the Elderly

BY

D. CORLESS

THE King Edward's Hospital Fund's 1965 report of an investigation into the dietary of elderly women living alone starts by stating "The precise nutritional needs of old people are unknown". Such is still the case today. Logically the subject may be divided into two headings: (1) overnutrition, and (2) undernutrition, with malnutrition affecting both groups. Nevertheless, though Sheldon noted that 20% of women over 80 were overweight, overnutrition can hardly be said to be a major problem in clinical geriatrics, even though it may produce sequelae such as atheromatous degeneration and osteoarthrosis.

The precise definition of both undernutrition and malnutrition become impossible if the normal nutritional needs are not known. Opinions vary widely about the incidence of malnutrition, particularly if subclinical malnutrition is looked for. Not surprisingly the incidence depends on the type of person investigated; thus it is lower in incidence among healthy people living at home than in enfeebled people in institutions. Geography has some bearing by reason of social factors, and the amount of sunlight and racial factors may also influence the incidence. Practising geriatrics in a predominantly working class area with a low retirement income, I find malnutrition in one form or another to be very common in hospital admissions.

SOCIAL, CLINICAL, AND ENVIRONMENTAL FACTORS

To consider diet in isolation could become an intellectual abstraction, for eating is not solely to sustain life: the preparation and consumption of food is done with others for enjoyment. Thus social isolation due to bereavement or families living some distance away plays a large part in malnutrition. Furthermore, depression in all its shades may be responsible for much self-neglect, while increasing physical infirmity leads to problems in shopping and cooking, compounded by poor housing and the isolation of houses from shops. Retirement to a "place near the sea" often brings unexpected difficulties when infirmities develop.

Illness in old age may lead to an inadequate diet, and it is important to remember that diseases of the gastrointestinal tract complicated by malabsorption may be asymptomatic. Very often the patient forgets to say that he has undergone a gastrectomy. Jejunal diverticula may

50

be found in patients with osteomalacia or vitamin B_{12} or folic acid deficiency. Idiopathic steatorrhoea can present in the elderly and blind-loop syndromes may also be seen. Drugs present an additional nutritional hazard and it is well known that barbiturates and anti-convulsants lead to folic acid deficiency. Not so widely recognized is that these drugs may precipitate osteomalacia because of an increased rate of breakdown of vitamin D metabolites.

Long-stay patients in institutions are often bereft of sunlight and have diets low in vitamin D and sometimes calcium. Thus, not sur-prisingly institutional osteomalacia may occur as well as scurvy, iron deficiency, and folate deficiency: 20% of patients recently admitted to hospital from the chronic sick institution were found to have biochemical osteomalacia.

THE IDEAL DIET

Longitudinal studies of the diet of old people show that there is an élite group whose nutrient intake is high and changes little with age. In others the nutrient intake declines probably owing to illnesses. The oft quoted "normal" decline in dietary intake after 80 is probably due to cross-sectional studies being used.

The total calorie intake needs to be related to energy expenditure, which is often quite low—even below 2,000 calories. Thus a reducing diet often has to be much lower than realized—600–800 calories, for instance.

The élite group referred to above was notable for having a high protein intake, 70 or more g per day; 58 or 60 g is the estimated need.

To provide 30% of the required number of calories would mean a fat content of 66 g for a 2,000 calorie diet and hence the normal intake of fat could vary from 50 to over 100 g.

Sixty per cent of the calorie requirements can be derived from carbohydrates, 266 g being needed for a 2,000 calorie diet.

The estimated vitamin needs are shown in table I.

TABLE I—*Daily Vitamin Needs for Elderly*

Vit. A	Vit. B_1	Vit. B_2	Vit. B_{12}	Folic Acid	Vit. C	Vit. D
5,000 I.U.	0·8 mg	1·3 mg	1 mg	250 µg	? 20 mg	?250 I.U.

The minimal quantity necessary of both vitamin C and D is not known accurately, and the limit of 20 mg of vitamin C may well be too low. 250 I.U. of vitamin D is an inspired guess and is half the daily need of a child.

The estimated daily mineral needs are probably 800 mg for calcium and 12 mg for iron. Cobalt, copper, magnesium, zinc, and other trace metals do not usually need to be considered by the clinician—though zinc depletion may delay wound healing.

CLINICAL PRESENTATION

Though it is more convenient to describe deficiency states one by one, deficiency states are usually compound problems; thus iron and folic acid deficiency, scurvy and osteomalacia may be found together.

Protein Deficiency

A lowered intake of protein leads to a loss of body weight, and equilibrium may be reached when the consequent weakness reduces energy expenditure. With severe protein lack the patient is apathetic, listless, and depressed, with pallor, hypothermia, and thin wrinkled skin. The eyes are sunken and all muscles are wasted. The temporal and masseter muscles seem to waste selectively in the early stages of protein deprivation. The pulse is slowed and the blood pressure lowered. Starvation oedema is dependent in type and not related solely to hypoproteinaemia. The body fat is lost. Occasionally old people are discovered in such a state. Milder degrees of this condition are usually encountered but, as always in geriatrics, it is difficult to decide between a change due to age and a mild clinical abnormality.

Fat and Carbohydrate Deficiencies

Rather than a specific fat deficiency it is much more likely that the patient suffers from other deficiencies if fat consumption falls—especially from lack of vitamin D. Often a falling fat intake is "balanced" by an increasing carbohydrate intake.

The undernourished have a diet with a high carbohydrate percentage as the carbohydrates are the cheapest form of food. Carbohydrate deficiency is therefore rare.

Vitamin Deficiencies

Vitamin A

Though some dietary surveys have shown a reduced intake of vitamin A there is no real evidence to demonstrate clinical signs of this. Vitamin A and carotenes are found in a wide variety of substances—dairy produce, fish oils, vegetables, and cereals—so that it is unlikely that a diet is completely deficient.

B Group

Vitamin B_1 (Thiamine).—Wet or dry beri-beri is the classical presentation of thiamine deprivation, and rarely this is seen in geriatric practice as high output cardiac failure with considerable oedema and a dilated heart; very occasionally the "dry" form with a peripheral neuritis affecting the legs, with burning paraesthesia, cramps, weakness, and tender calves, is encountered. Biochemical evidence of thiamine deficiency has been found in a large percentage of long-stay patients.

Vitamin B₂ (Riboflavine) and Nicotinic Acid.—Deficiency of both these vitamins is shown by abnormalities of the mouth and tongue, skin, and muscles. Nicotinic acid deficiency may be complicated by diarrhoea, peripheral neuritis, and mental changes. Cheilosis, angular stomatitis, and glossitis may have causes other than riboflavine deficiency —for example, iron deficiency or ill fitting dentures—and hence these signs must be interpreted cautiously. Nasolabial seborrhoea (that is, enlarged, often red follicles near the sides of the nose with follicles plugged with dry sebaceous material) occurs with riboflavine deficiency.

The blood riboflavine level may be estimated, but often does not correlate with the clinical state even if the signs of riboflavine deficiency are classical. The evidence is also conflicting about whether the signs respond to vitamin therapy.

Folic Acid.—Nutritional folic acid deficiency is common among old people, though a macrocytic anaemia due to this is much less common. Serum folic acid levels below 2 mμg/100 ml probably indicate deficiency but the red cell folate level is now thought to be a better guide. Gastrointestinal lesions should be sought and a careful inquiry into drugs prescribed should be made.

Vitamin B₁₂.—Atrophic gastritis occurs increasingly with age and the incidence of pernicious anaemia increases also; a pure dietary cause for B_{12} deficiency is rare. When the classical features of pernicious anaemia are present, diagnosis presents no difficulty. Neurological manifestations may occur without anaemia, and dementia with low levels of vitamin B_{12} in the cerebrospinal fluid and normal levels in the serum has been described in the elderly.

Vitamin C

Severe scurvy is sometimes seen but lesser degrees are more difficult to spot. Hyperkeratosis of the hair follicles causes the hair to curl within the plaque of keratin (Royston's curls) and these are numerous over the anterior abdominal wall (they occur normally over pressure sites). Haemorrhage occurs around the hair follicle and petechial haemorrhages appear especially around the ankles and feet. Large spontaneous ecchymoses appear in muscles and skin, and haemarthroses may also occur. Gingivitis does not occur in the edentulous.

Scurvy tends to affect those who cannot cook (widowers) and those who have bizarre diets—for example, prolonged gastric diets. The most useful test is the white cell ascorbic acid level (normal > 2 mg/100 ml).

In conditions of "stress" such as a healing bed sore, vitamin C requirements may increase and supplementation is necessary. Patients in institutions are highly vulnerable. Mass catering destroys vitamin C, so that not only may the basic diet be deficient but a plentiful supply of fresh fruit may not be provided.

Vitamin D

The diagnosis of severe osteomalacia is easy provided that the doctor thinks of it. Backache, bone pains, fractures, and muscular weakness of a proximal myopathy type with the finding of Chvostek's and/or Trousseau's signs are the main clinical findings. Demonstration of Looser's zones radiologically and the finding of low levels of serum calcium and phosphorus, and a high level of alkaline phosphatase, confirms the diagnosis. The histological appearance of a bone biopsy specimen is more difficult to interpret in a severely osteoporotic skeleton.

TABLE II—*Some Dietary Supplements Available* (*Contents per* 100 g.)

Product	Calories	Protein (g)	Fat (g)	Carbo-hydrates (g)	Vit. A (I.U.)	Vit. B (mg)
Carnation (Instant Breakfast)	357	21·8	2·59	61·6	4,090	1 5
Casilan	344	90	1·8	—	—	—
Forceval	370	55	<19	30	8,333	10

Product	Ribo-flavine (mg)	Folic acid (μg)	Vit. C (mg)	Vit. D (I.U.)	Iron (mg)	Calcium (mg)
Carnation (Instant Breakfast)	2·6	—	76	—	10	—
Casilan	—	—	—	—	—	1,130
Forceval	6·6	0·03	170	850	17	1,170

The biochemical findings may be normal in patients with histologically proved osteomalacia, and a low alkaline phosphatase level occurs in patients with osteomalacia who are bed-fast. Subclinical states are very difficult to identify and the relatively high incidence of raised alkaline phosphatase levels in patients with skeletal rarefaction may be an indication that a mild degree of osteomalacia is more common than realized. The fact that some elderly people and long-stay patients have low vitamin D intake (often below 50 I.U. daily) and are confined to the home or an institution without access to sunlight should make the doctor particularly mindful of osteomalacia. Thus measurements of the serum calcium, phosphorus, alkaline phosphatase, and serum protein levels should be part of every elderly patient's screening procedure.

Mineral Deficiencies

Calcium

There is no evidence that calcium deficiency leads to osteoporosis or that a low calcium intake is associated with any clinical state. A low calcium intake is dangerous if vitamin D preparations are given as it may worsen the hypocalcaemia with the development of tetany and cardiac arrest.

Iron

Iron-deficiency anaemia is common in the elderly owing to a low intake (especially in long-stay patients), poor absorption due to several factors, and gastrointestinal blood loss from hiatus hernia or diverticulitis. It is always difficult to examine thoroughly the gastrointestinal tract of a patient with iron deficiency anaemia.

MANAGEMENT OF UNDERNUTRITION

It is most important to identify the underlying cause of undernutrition seen in the elderly—including depression, dementia, physical incapacity, low income, bereavement, "therapy"—and to exclude any underlying disease causing anorexia or malabsorption. Very often the situation may be improved by general measures such as a supplementary pension, a home help, or meals-on-wheels. Rehousing, especially sheltered housing, can help greatly. An institution is a last resort, but this is not without its own dangers.

Without doubt the best treatment is preventative, and good dietary advice should and does form part of pre-retirement education. With established malnutrition the best treatment is still a good diet. During the initial phase protein, vitamin, and mineral supplements may be used, and several are now available which are very palatable (table II). Iron therapy often needs to be given separately, as does vitamin C and D therapy. Nevertheless, since pills and capsules are not consumed reliably by many patients their number is best kept to a minimum.

The patient who will not eat and visibly fades away is fortunately an infrequent problem. It can be difficult to decide how energetic the treatment should be and an intubated patient struggling to die needs a humane approach. Adding life to years and not years to life should always be the guideline of therapy.

BIBLIOGRAPHY

Baker, A. Z., *Gerontologia Clinica*, 1962, **4**, 100.

Brocklehurst, J. C., Griffiths, L. L., Taylor, G. F., Marks, J., Scott, D. L., and Blackley J., *Gerontologia Clinica*, 1968, **10**, 309.

Exton-Smith, A. N., and Stanton, B. R., *Report of an Investigation into the Dietary of Elderly Women Living Alone*. London, King Edward's Hospital Fund for London, 1965.

Exton-Smith, A. N., and Stanton, B. R., *A Longitudinal Study of the Dietary of Elderly Women*. London, King Edward's Hospital Fund for London, 1970.

Exton-Smith, A. N., Hodkinson, H. M., and Stanton, B. R., *Lancet*, 1966, **2**, 999.

Hodkinson, A. M., Stanton, B. R., Round, P., and Morgan, C., *Lancet*, 1973, **1**, 910.

McLennan, W. J., Caird, F. I., and Macleod, C. C., *Age and Ageing*, 1972, **1**, 131.

Macleod, R. D. M., *Age and Ageing*, 1972, **1**, 99.

Role of Day Hospital Care

BY

J. C. BROCKLEHURST

GERIATRIC medicine initiated an early form of progressive patient care in hospital—through acute admission ward, to rehabilitation ward, and continuing care ward. The geriatric day hospital is a logical extension of this system and forms a bridge between the hospital and the community. The ever-increasing numbers and proportion of elderly people, particular the very old, in our society inevitably increase the incidence of disabling disease. The provision of day care for the treatment and support of elderly disabled people has been an attempt, attended with a good deal of success, to prevent the admission to hospital of more and more of these old people.

SOCIAL DAY CARE

Day care for the elderly includes a wide variety of social and hospital provisions which must be clearly distinguished. Social day care is provided either by local authorities or by voluntary organizations (for example, old peoples welfare committees)—or occasionally by thoughtful employers. Social day care itself offers a whole spectrum of facilities.[1] Anderson's definition of social day care is as follows: "Clubs and social centres exist for all old people, to increase social contact and to give scope and facilities for new pursuits in retirement".

Several main types of day care are now available. Day care centres, most usually instituted by local authorities, provide a substantial amount of personal care to at least a small proportion of clients. Referral is usually through general practitioners or social workers. There are a wide range of services, including bathing, chiropody, meals, and provision of low priced foods. Psychogeriatric day care centres are similar to day care centres but require a greater degree of supervision. Their purpose is more that of a crèche than a club. Since it is now the Department of Health and Social Security's policy to support old people suffering from dementia, who are neither physically handicapped nor pose behavioural problems, in the community, the importance of psychogeriatric day care centres is likely to increase.[2]

Both these types of social day centres may be provided by local authorities under the 1968 Health Services and Public Health Act and both require transport to bring the clients to them.

Social centres or social clubs come in many varieties; some are open

57

seven days a week, others only one half day a fortnight. They usually have a regular membership and are often organized by the retired people themselves. Shelters (rest centre or drop-in) may be provided by local communities or employers and serve simply as a communal meeting place which elderly people may use as they wish.

Communal rooms in sheltered housing and other housing schemes clearly offer a great opportunity for day care, in which both residents in the sheltered housing and other people living in the area may join together. A most important development for the future will be the provision of a restaurant so that residents in sheltered housing may have at least one communal cooked meal a day, where they may be joined by elderly people from the local community.

Lunch clubs are an important and desirable alternative to meals-on-wheels. Work centres may be provided either by the local authority, commercial organizations, or voluntary bodies. Essentially, retired people come here to engage in productive work for which they are paid. This has, of course, very important social and emotional advantages.

These various types of social day care available at present must be clearly distinguished from the geriatric day hospital.

DAY HOSPITALS

Day hospitals are part of the hospital service and are generally situated within a district general hospital in close relationship to the geriatric rehabilitation department. In many cases, day hospital and geriatric rehabilitation department share the same premises and facilities. This is a particularly desirable concept, which allows patients who have been undergoing rehabilitation to return to their homes and yet have the security of a continuing contact with the hospital and so with their therapists, until they are firmly settled back at home. Though day hospitals have many uses other than this, this is one of the most important, and one which guards against waste of hospital resources.

The concept of a geriatric day hospital must now be extended to include the psychogeriatric day hospital. Though not many are so far available it is part of the clearly defined policy of the Department of Health and Social Security to provide two places per 1,000 people over 65 for geriatric day hospital care and an additional two places per 1,000 people over 65 for psychogeriatric day hospital care. The psychogeriatric day hospital may be established adjoining the geriatric day hospital and share several facilities. Alternatively, and hitherto more commonly, it may be set up within a psychiatric hospital, though in future, of course, these will be replaced. A further possibility is that the psychogeriatric day hospital may be situated within the community hospital or general-practitioner hospital, particularly in rural areas.

Development

Geriatric day hospitals first developed from occupational therapy departments. The first purpose-built geriatric day hospital was opened in Oxford at Cowley Road Hospital, and this has served as the model for subsequent development. The day hospital at Oxford was opened in 1958 and by the end of 1970 there were 120 geriatric day hospitals in the UK. Now most geriatric departments include a day hospital, and increasingly purpose-built day hospitals are superseding adaptations of various other hospital premises.

Work

Elderly patients come to a day hospital for one of four main reasons: rehabilitation; maintenance treatment; medical or nursing investigation; or social care.

Rehabilitation is an important part of geriatric practice since so often the problem is one of physical disability: there is prospect of improvement, though often not of recovery. It is helpful to see re-habilitation as a finite process to which there is usually an end—reached when the patient achieves his maximum degree of independence.

Maintenance treatment is important in old age since having once achieved maximum independence many elderly people will deteriorate slowly (and sometimes quite rapidly) once they are cut off from the stimulus of the geriatric rehabilitation department. Much important and laborious work can thereby be undone, particularly if relatives are over-protective or the old person poorly motivated. Once-weekly day hospital attendance perhaps for an indefinite period often ensures that the state of independence achieved is maintained.

Medical and nursing procedures in the day hospital form a very variable part of current geriatric practice. In a few departments great stress is laid on these;[3] in most some use is made of the day hospital for procedures such as sternal marrow punctures, the supervision and treatment of faecal incontinence, glucose tolerance tests, etc. On the other hand, obviously it is not appropriate to bring elderly people up to a day hospital simply to carry out procedures which might equally well be done by the district nurse or the family doctor in the patient's home.

The distinction between social day care and the geriatric day hospital has already been emphasized, but a few elderly people are so physically disabled as to be unsuitable for social day centres and yet have needs for companionship and relief of their isolation. Its nursing care makes geriatric day hospital the appropriate place for such patients. In some day hospitals severely disabled younger patients are brought for this purpose. Another, if uncommon, aspect of social care is when a disabled elderly patient may be discharged home from hospital and looked after at night and at the weekend, but when the relative on whom he depends has to work. Discharge may then be possible only if day hospital attendance can be arranged.

Patients

In a national survey of day hospitals Brocklehurst[4] found that consultant geriatricians placed most importance on physical rehabilitation and physical maintenance (89% and 78%, respectively of respondents). Half laid stress on the social care of physically disabled people as important, 36% on medical or nursing procedures, and 21% on the social care of mentally confused old people. In a more detailed survey of five day hospitals the numbers of patients actually attending for these various purposes were as follows: rehabilitation 27%, physical maintenance 42%, social reason 26%, and other 5%.

This survey also noted the source of referral of 465 day hospital patients as follows: in-patient geriatric ward 32%, medical ward 7%, other wards 2%, geriatric outpatient consultative clinic 29%, domiciliary or assessment visit 13%, and by direct negotiation with the general practitioner 17%. Most people attending the day hospitals surveyed were aged between 75 and 84 and the major diagnostic categories were stroke (30%) and arthritis (26%).

Staff

The day hospital should be regarded as a ward within the hospital —in fact, Andrews has suggested that it should be called a day ward rather than a day hospital. This emphasizes that staffing should be on similar levels of that of an inpatient ward and that management should be along similar lines. The day hospital is generally in charge of the consultant geriatrician and consists of three main departments—nursing, physiotherapy, and occupational therapy—with a smaller involvement of speech therapists, social workers, volunteers, and administrators. A doctor must attend daily to maintain records and to initiate investigation and treatment of patients. There should also be a case conference of the whole medical, social, and therapeutic team at least once weekly to review the patients' progress. To be dynamic a day hospital must be continually discharging and accepting new patients and there should never be a waiting list. It is a great advantage if there are clear pathways between the day hospital and the various social day care facilities so that those who no longer need the therapeutic aspect of day care may continue to enjoy its social benefit.

Advantages

The advantages of the geriatric day hospital lie first in allowing the treatment of many elderly people without hospital admission, particularly when outpatient attendance at a physiotherapy department would be unsuitable. The need is for a continuing therapeutic environment where the pace is slower but activity continues throughout most of the day. The day hospital also allows the earlier discharge of patients and their subsequent supervision until they are safely settled at home. Another advantage is that the hours are attractive to staff and recruitment of suitable staff is often easier than to the inpatient wards.

Problems

Day hospitals are not without their problems. Probably the greatest of these lies in the provision of ambulance transport. It is exceptional for any patient needing day hospital treatment to be able to come independently. A few can be brought by relatives in cars, and in the occasional area taxis are hired for this purpose, but generally day hospitals must depend on the ambulance service for the delivery and returning home of their patient. This requires special and appropriate transport—for example, a vehicle with eight to ten seats with a hydraulic or other lift, good visibility for the passengers, safe seating, and good heating. Such a vehicle is likely to take between an hour and an hour and a half to collect its complement of patients and so those collected first may well spend upwards of an hour in the vehicle. For most of them this is of no hardship provided that the vehicle is appropriate, since it is likely to be the only time that they get out of their own homes.

It is essential that ambulances should bring patients to the day hospital and take them home according to a pre-arranged time-table and that vehicles are not used which are apt to be diverted for other purposes. The whole professional team in the day hospital awaits the arrival of the patients and if ambulance services are erratic there is an enormous waste of these professional resources. It is equally frustrating for the old person sitting for two or three hours awaiting the ambulance's arrival. Furthermore, patients coming to day hospitals are often relying on this as their only source of food that day, and perhaps of heating and other care. If the ambulance does not collect them they may suffer great hardship, as was shown in a survey of the effect of industrial action by the ambulance service on day hospital patients.[5]

Finally, what of the future ? The day hospital is now firmly established and in due course every geriatric department will have one as an essential part of its service. There may be an increase of specialization within day hospitals, some developing more as day wards for medical and nursing treatment, others becoming the local stroke rehabilitation unit or orthopaedic rehabilitation unit for elderly people. Possibly some smaller day hospitals may be set up in association with community hospitals, where the emphasis will be on maintenance and social treatment. The day hospital serves as an excellent focus bringing together community medical care (the general-practitioner team) and the geriatric hospital team. The day hospital is in many ways a shop window for the geriatric service and undoubtedly a good one adds immeasurably to the morale of the whole geriatric department.

REFERENCES

[1] Anderson, D. C., *Report on Leisure and Day Care Facilities for the Old*. London, Age Concern, 1972.

[2] Davidge, J. L., in *The Elderly Mind*, London, British Hospital Journal/ Hospital International, 1972.

[3] Andrews, J., Fairley, A., Hyland, M., *Journal of the American Geriatrics Society*, 1970, **18**, 378.

[4] Brocklehurst, J. C., *The Geriatric Day Hospital*, London, King Edward's Hospital Fund for London, 1970.

[5] Prinsley, D. N., *British Medical Journal*, 1971, **3**, 170.

Anaemia in the Elderly

BY

J. H. THOMAS

ANAEMIA is always pathological and the clinical impression of its presence or absence often erroneous; it is not a concomitant of ageing. The reported incidence has varied greatly. Pincherle and Shanks[1] found it in only 0·42% of 2,000 business executives, 300 of whom were over 60 years. On the other hand, Parsons and his colleagues,[2] in a community survey, found an incidence of 7·2% in men and 11·1% in women in the age group 65–74 years, and in 20·8% and 23·3% respectively in those who were older. The Health Department's Nutritional Panel[3] gave a figure of 7·3%, which was about the same for men and women. The incidence among hospital admissions is about 30%.

The following groups of old people are particularly at risk of developing anaemia: those living alone, with mental deterioration, with apathy or depression, over 75 years of age, with diminished mobility, who have had gastric surgery, and who have been anaemic in the past.

CAUSES

Occult bleeding from the gastrointestinal tract is a frequent cause, but others—including insufficient intake of nutrients, diminished absorption, and general disease—are also important. Contributory factors, such as atrophic gastritis, chronic infection, carcinoma, renal disease, and the development of antibodies may also be present, and several factors may operate simultaneously.

Red cells from the marrow circulate for about 120 days and are then destroyed by the reticuloendothelial system, their iron and globin being reutilized. Derangement at any stage leads to anaemia.

TYPES OF ANAEMIA

The deficiency anaemias are of paramount importance and may be classified according to the deficient haemopoietic factor.

Iron-deficiency Anaemia

Iron-deficiency anaemia is the most common type. Haemoglobin formation is diminished, resulting in hypochromia with a low mean corpuscular haemoglobin concentration of 32 % or less. The red cells are usually smaller than normal. There is sideropenia and reduction of iron saturation to below 16%, a level below 10% being pathognomonic.[4] Marrow smear and sections have a diminished iron content.

In iron-deficiency anaemia due to blood loss the latter has usually occurred from the gastrointestinal tract, and occult blood testing of the stools is mandatory in every anaemic patient. When repeat tests are positive x-ray investigation of the gastrointestinal tract is necessary, provided the bleeding is not due to such causes as thrombocytopenia or a raised blood urea. Microscopic examination of the urine should also be part of routine investigations.

Vitamin B_{12}-deficiency Anaemia

In vitamin B_{12} deficiency red cell formation is defective. Macrocytes appear in the peripheral blood, and the marrow becomes megaloblastic.

The serum B_{12} value is below 111 pg per ml, and usually considerably so. (It is important to remember that if a bacillary method is used for estimating this level antibiotic therapy, particularly of ampicillin, should have been discontinued for at least three days, as otherwise a false low value may be obtained).

Nevertheless, a low serum vitamin B_{12} value can be obtained when the peripheral red cell is normal or hypochromic. Findings in pernicious anaemia include achlorhydria and improvement in vitamin B_{12} absorption when it is combined with intrinsic factor. Gastric parietal cell antibodies (IgG) are present in 80% and intrinsic factor antibodies (IgA) in 50% of cases. The incidence is around 7 per 1,000, though it is higher in those with rheumatoid arthritis or hypothyroidism. There is a familial pattern. Other reasons for vitamin B_{12} deficiency are partial gastrectomy, malnutrition, ileal malabsorption, and increased utilization of the vitamin by proliferating organisms in jejunal or duodenal diverticula.

Folate Deficiency

Folate deficiency may be due to malnutrition; malabsorption from jejunal disease; secondary to drugs, particularly those used in epilepsy; increased utilization, as in myelofibrosis; or excess loss, as in exfoliative dermatitis. The full clinical picture should be evaluated before a certain diagnosis is made. Measurement of the faecal fat may be necessary, and also x-ray examination of the small intestine. Its incidence increases with age, presumably owing to dietary difficulties.

In folate deficiency the fully developed blood picture is indistinguishable from that produced by vitamin-B_{12} deficiency, as the two factors are interrelated. The serum folate value is below 2·5 ng per ml and the red cell value less than 140 ng per ml of packed red cells; but this latter measurement is a poor guide when there is associated vitamin B_{12} deficiency.

Other Deficiencies

In vitamin C deficiency the cells are normocytic though an occasional macrocyte may be seen. In deficiency of vitamin B_6 (pyridoxine) there is hypochromia with a low mean corpuscular haemoglobin concentration, because the utilization of iron by the red cells is impaired.

Mixed Deficiencies

Mixed deficiences are common, and are pinpointed when the various serum values are determined in all anaemic patients. The cells may be dimorphic or normocytic, but no appearance excludes the diagnosis.

"Marrow" Anaemia

True aplasia is unusual, but relative marrow failure is fairly common. There is mild normocytic normochromic anaemia with a poor marrow response. The cause has not been elucidated, though it is probably multifactorial. Infiltration with fibrous, myelomatous, or neoplastic tissue may result in a leucoerythroblastic picture, which is characterized by a leucocytosis and a mixture of immature red and white blood cells.

Haemolytic Anaemia

The overt type of haemolytic anaemia, due to increased fragility of the red cells or damage by toxins, drugs, or antibodies, is less common than the latent variety. In this variant the red cell life is reduced, though not enough to produce anaemia if the marrow is functioning normally. Defects in both the peripheral cells and the bone marrow may be present in renal failure, liver dysfunction, carcinoma, and terminal disease.

PRESENTATION OF ANAEMIAS

When anaemia is of rapid onset there is weakness, shortness of breath, and giddiness, but when it develops slowly, as it usually does, the symptoms are often ascribed to ageing. Mental changes, angina pectoris, or heart failure may all be the presenting features, together with apathy, depression, or diminished mobility. The overall picture can be one of multiple lesions, with the anaemia being part of a wide spectrum of diseases.

In making the diagnosis a full history must be taken, paying special attention to the social environment, mental state, and mobility. Diet and mastication should be assessed, and also bowel action. Previous surgery or anaemia should be noted. The physical examination must be complete as no system can be neglected for a possible cause. The sequence followed in the investigations depends a great deal on the clinical features. Laboratory tests are necessary. It is helpful for the family doctor if the advice of a physician or pathologist is readily available, together with an open door to the pathology department. The tests that are necessary are directed towards the clarification of formation, destruction, and loss of the red blood cells.

TREATMENT OF DEFICIENCY ANAEMIAS

Iron Deficiency

About 200 mg of elemental iron are given daily between meals, and the same dosage continued for at least six months after the haemoglobin has reached normal levels, to replenish the body stores. If intake is unreliable the calculated deficiency may be corrected by intramuscular therapy.

Vitamin B_{12}

One thousand μg is given weekly for four doses and then three-monthly, unless there is renal or hepatic disease when the same dosage is given two-monthly, owing to increased body turnover.[5] The reticulocytosis should reach its highest level by the seventh day. If the cell count is one million the injection should give rise to a reticulocytosis of 40% of the red cells, while with one of three million the response should be 10%. Hydroxocobalamin is preferable to cyanocobalamin, and life-long injections are necessary in pernicious anaemia, ileal malabsorption, and when dietary inadequacy cannot be corrected. Care is also necessary to ensure that iron or folate deficiency, or both, does not develop.

Folate Deficiency

Five milligrammes of folate three times a day are given until the blood count is satisfactory, and then the dose is reduced to five mg daily. The body stores of vitamin B_{12} must be normal as otherwise neurological complications develop. When the diagnosis is in doubt a cover dose of 500 μg B_{12} should be given three-monthly, or the vitamin B_{12} serum level should be confirmed as being normal every six months. Only when there is a continued cause for the deficiency, such as malabsorption or antiepileptic therapy, need long-term treatment be given.

Blood Transfusion

Whole blood is necessary when there is acute blood loss, but otherwise, haematinic therapy usually suffices. Sometimes, however, packed red cells, 400 ml or thereabouts, repeated if necessary, may be life saving when the severity of the anaemia has caused heart failure, mental confusion, or extreme apathy. Patients with aplastic anaemia have to be transfused regularly, and the procedure is often necessary when urgent surgery is contemplated, or when early radiological investigation of the gastrointestinal tract is essential.

MANAGEMENT

The advisability or otherwise of home management depends on the degree of illness, the extent and type of anaemia, the availability of the hospital service, and the social circumstances of the patient. Several questions arise: Is the anaemia due to a primary blood disorder, such as leukaemia? Is it secondary to malnutrition, malabsorption, blood loss, drug therapy, or general disease? Is it separate from the other abnormalities that may be present? Most of the answers are obtained by studying the haemoglobin level, the blood film, and the absolute values; by taking a careful history paying particular attention to food intake; and by carrying out a detailed physical examination, noting the presence or absence of adenopathy, splenomegaly, purpura, and the tell-tale signs of malnutrition, chronic infection, or carcinoma. Occult blood testing of the stools is necessary, and if the anaemia is refractory or the cause obscure, consideration given to the possible presence of hypoplasia or haemolysis. The level of blood urea may supply the answer.

Whenever suitable the treatment should be at home, but the anaemia should never be dismissed as an incidental finding, of little or no consequence, because the underlying cause may be of vital significance. Ideally, the serum values of iron, vitamin B_{12}, and folate should be obtained despite the complexity of their interrelationship; but it is justifiable to give all three haematinics as an emergency when the patient is seriously ill—though future management is simplified if a blood sample is taken beforehand.

PREVENTION

Anaemia has a high morbidity and therefore every effort should be made to reduce its incidence. Two methods are practicable. Firstly, primary prevention, by ensuring that all elderly people receive adequate quantities of protein and of haemopoietic factors in their daily diet—that is, 10-12 mg iron, 10 μg B_{12}, 100 μg folate, 35 mg vitamin C, and 2 mg pyridoxine. Ignorance, poverty, prejudice, apathy, and isolation are some of the resisting forces. The other method is secondary prevention—by detecting and treating the early case, (that is, when the haemoglobin level is around 11·6 g per 100 ml) and thereby prevent, or delay, progression. Regular home visiting by doctors or nurses, or both, is essential, and special attention should be paid to those at risk.[6]

REFERENCES

[1] Picherele, G., and Shanks, J., *British Journal of Social and Preventive Medicine*, 1967, **21**, 40.

[2] Kilpatrick G. S., Parsons, P. L., and Withey, J. L., *Practitioner*, 1965, **195**, 656.

[3] *A Nutrition Survey of the Elderly*, Reports on Health and Social Subjects, No. 3, p. 57. London, H.M.S.O., 1972.

[4] Wintrobe, M. M., *Clinical Haematology*, 6th ed., p. 597. London, Kimpton, 1967.

[5] Adams, J. F., and Boddy, K., *The Cobalamins*, A Glaxo Symposium, p. 166. ed. H. R. V. Arnstein and R. J. Wrighton. Edinburgh and London, Churchill Livingstone, 1971.

[6] Thomas, J. H., and Powell, D. E. B., *Blood Disorders in the Elderly*, p. 133 Bristol, Wright, 1971.

Problems of Interpretation of Laboratory Findings in the Old

BY

F. I. CAIRD

HAEMATOLOGICAL, biochemical, and endocrine disorders are common in old age, and are often eminently remediable, but assessment of their significance is frequently hampered by problems of interpretation of the laboratory data on which the diagnosis and management of such disorders usually rest. There are several reasons for these difficulties in interpretation. Simple lack of knowledge of well-established normal values is not infrequent. Many normal values in the elderly are identical to those recognized for the young. If an abnormal value is mistakenly considered to be normal "for the patient's age," the opportunity for correct diagnosis and active treatment will be missed. Conversely some normal values differ in the elderly from those taught for the young. If a value normal for the patient's age is considered abnormal, then the patient may be subjected to unnecessary and possibly even hazardous further investigations—or an incorrect diagnosis and so perhaps prognosis will result. In both instances the necessary information may be found in journals which are not easily accessible, may not yet be in the textbooks, and in consequence is not taught.

A further difficulty arises from the fact that some normal values are not yet certainly established for the elderly. One reason for this is the high frequency of disease states in old age, which may make distinction of normal from abnormal uncertain. There is often in addition a problem in assessing the significance of minor deviations from normality as shown by laboratory tests in old people, and consequent difficulty in management of patients with such abnormalities.

The present paper attempts to review and discuss in respect of the elderly several commonly performed laboratory tests and the problems of interpretation which they present, both in relation to screening procedures and to the assessment of sick old people.

HAEMATOLOGICAL TESTS

Haemoglobin Concentration

The haemoglobin concentration does not change significantly with age,[1] and thus values considered to indicate anaemia should be identical in young and old. If a haemoglobin concentration of less than 12 g/100 ml is taken to define anaemia,[2] or at least as an indication for further

69

investigation, a few elderly women will be found whose haemoglobin concentration lies between 11·5 and 11·9 g/100 ml, yet who have no evident cause for anaemia;[3] and several men will be overlooked, whose haemoglobin concentration is above 12 g/100 ml, yet who have a definite and diagnosable abnormality remediable by treatment. Nevertheless, 12 g/100 ml is probably the best single level for the definition of anaemia in old age.

The standard haematological indices (PCV, MCH, MCHC, MCV) are unaffected by age, and so are the appearances of the blood film. A low MCHC and hypochromia should thus be taken to indicate iron deficiency, at least in the first instance, since this is the commonest single cause of anaemia in old age.[3 4] Similarly a high MCV and macrocytosis are evidence of the need to exclude a megaloblastic state due to deficiency of vitamin B_{12} or folate.

Serum Iron Levels

The serum iron tends to fall with age,[5 6] so that levels as low as 50 μg/100 ml may be found when iron stores are adequate, as shown by the presence of substantial amounts in the bone marrow. The iron-binding saturation (serum iron as a percentage of total iron-binding capacity (TIBC) is a more reliable index, since probably levels of 16% or below are not found when there are more than traces of iron in the bone marrow.[7 8] Higher saturations may on occasion accompany undoubted iron deficiency, and the MCHC and blood film should always be taken into account. As many as 10% of elderly people living at home may have an abnormally low iron-binding saturation, but a normal haemoglobin concentration and a normal blood film.[3] There is evidence that women of reproductive age who show a similar picture have a high chance of developing frank iron-deficiency anaemia within a few years,[9] but whether the same is true of the elderly is not known. Since no symptomatic benefit accrues from the treatment of such people with iron,[10 11] there is at present no reason to treat such people with what has been termed "sideropenia without anaemia".

Folate and B_{12} Levels

Somewhat similar difficulties arise in the interpretation of serum folate levels in the elderly. Values as low as 1·5 ng/ml are often found in the absence of anaemia or neurological disorder.[3 4] Again, there is no information about the prognostic significance of such levels, which would be considered abnormal in youth or middle age. A low serum vitamin B_{12} level (below 140 pg/ml) can be taken to indicate deficiency of that vitamin as a cause of a megaloblastic anaemia in an old person, but low levels are also not uncommonly encountered in elderly people without anaemia, macrocytosis, or disorder of the nervous system.[3] It is not yet known how frequently or how soon overt clinical disease may be expected to develop in such people, who may perhaps still possess hepatic stores of vitamin B_{12} sufficient to last for long periods, but it is known that they are not benefited, in term of symptoms, from vitamin B_{12} therapy.[12]

White Cell Count

The white cell count tends to fall with age, mainly owing to a reduction in lymphocyte count. Table I gives values derived from a study of 480 old people living at home.[14] The upper limit of normal for the total white cell count is shown to be 9,000/mm³, which is less than the textbook figure of 10–11,000/mm³. Total counts over 9,000/mm³ may thus be taken to indicate leucocytosis. The lower limit of the total count is 3,000/mm³, and leucopenia should therefore not be diagnosed unless the count is below this figure, rather than the customary levels of 4–5,000/mm³. These two conclusions are good examples of the need for accurate knowledge of normal values in old age, to ensure correct diagnosis where this is appropriate, and to avoid unnecessary further investigation.

TABLE I—*Range of Normal Values for the Leucocyte Count in People over 65 Years of Age*[14]

	Absolute Count (cells/mm³)	Differential Count (%)
Total	3,100–8,900	—
Polymorphs	1,800–6,500	45–85
Lymphocytes	700–3,500	10–50
Eosinophils	—	0–8
Monocytes	—	0–8

ESR

Some uncertainty surrounds the interpretation of the erythrocyte sedimentation rate (ESR) in old age. Studies to determine the true normal limits of this valuable simple test are difficult to carry out in the elderly, since even after the exclusion of acutely ill subjects, who constitute a high proportion of any hospital series, there remain many people with chronic conditions associated with an elevation of the ESR. Undoubtedly mean values rise steadily with age in healthy people, and are higher in women than men,[15] and it is also clear that no convincing cause may be found in old people for values as high as 35–40 mm/hr.[16 17] As in younger people, the isolated finding of a raised ESR is best repeated after a few weeks, and only a persistent rise outside the limits mentioned should be regarded as an indication for further investigation.

BIOCHEMICAL TESTS

In many commonly performed biochemical tests mean normal values and the range encountered in relatively healthy old people are identical to those found in the young (table II). Abnormalities in these cannot therefore be attributed to ageing, but require assessment and diagnosis. The abnormalities most frequently met with are hypokalaemia,[19] of which the commonest cause is diuretic drugs, and hypoalbuminaemia, which may be due to chronic infection, diffuse liver disease, or less often to simple malnutrition. The criteria for the identification of these abnormalities, and the action which should follow their detection, do not differ in essence in old age from standard practice in younger patients.

TABLE II—*Normal Values for Biochemical Measurements in Old Age*[18]

Measurement		Units	Mean ± SD	Range
Na+		m/Eql	141 ± 3	135–146
K+		,,	4·4 ± 0·4	3·6–5·2
Cl		,,	102 ± 3	96–108
HCO₃		,,	25 ± 3	19–31
Total Protein		g/100 ml	7·1 ± 5	6·1–8·1
Albumin		,,	4·1 ± 0·4	3·3–4·9
Globulin		,,	3·1 ± 0·5	2·1–4·1
Mg++		mg/100 ml	2·0 ± 0·25	1·5–2·5
PO₄	M	,,	3·1 ± 0·5	2·1–4·1
	F	,,	3·4 ± 0·6	2·2–4·6
Bilirubin		,,	*	0·3–1·5

* Lognormal frequency distribution.

Blood Urea and Creatinine

For a second group of measurements the range of normal values is not the same in the elderly as in the young (table III). The most obvious example is the blood urea, which is the result of the body's production of the urea and the glomerular filtration rate. The former probably falls with age, and the latter certainly does,[20] and to a greater extent, so that the plasma concentration of urea rises with age.[21 23] The upper limit of normal for the blood urea in people over 65 is about 60 mg/100 ml.[24] Renal failure, with its poor prognosis and attendant potentially hazardous investigations, should not be diagnosed if the blood urea is below this figure. Exactly similar considerations apply to the serum creatinine, for which a reasonable upper limit of normal in old age is 1·9 mg/100 ml, rather than the customary figure of 1·6 mg/100 ml.

TABLE III—*Normal Values which differ in Old Age*[18]

Substance		Units	Mean ± SD	Range
Urea		mg/100 ml	*	22–60
Creatinine		,,	*	0·4–1·9
Cholesterol	M	,,	*	160–345
.. ..	F	,,	*	180–435
Ca++	M	,,	9·5 ± 0·5	8·5–10·5
.. ..	F	,,	9·8 ± 0·5	8·7–10·7
Uric acid	M	,,	5·5 ± 1·2	3·1–7·9
.. ..	F	,,	4·9 ± 1·4	2·1–7·7
Alkaline phosphatase		K-A units	*	5–20

* Lognormal frequency distribution.

Uric Acid, Cholesterol, and Calcium Levels

An age-related rise in serum uric acid is well-documented.[25] [26] Levels below 7·7 mg/100 ml should be regarded as normal (table III), and cannot be used to support a diagnosis of gout in an old person. The thiazide diuretics are the commonest cause of a rise of the serum uric acid level in old age.

The serum cholesterol concentration rises with age, and after the menopause is higher in women than in men, the reverse of the situation below that age.[26] [27] There may well be considerable local variation in normal levels in old age, associated with nutritional differences,[28] but in urban Scotland over 40% of women and 8% of men over the age of 65 have a serum cholesterol level of over 300 mg/100 ml.[18] (Fig. 1). These high values are not associated with coronary artery disease,[29] or with hypothyroidism, and only very high figures (of over 450 mg/ 100 ml or so) can be used to support the latter diagnosis in an old person. There is no evidence that lowering the serum cholesterol is of benefit to an elderly patient.

A further example of a normal range which may differ in old people is provided by the serum calcium. There seems little doubt that in elderly women the commonly accepted upper limit of 10·5 mg/100 ml is too low,[18] [26] and that values of 10·7 or even 11·0 mg/100 ml may be found in the absence of any symptoms or other biochemical or radiological evidence of hyperparathyroidism or other cause of hypercalcaemia. The sex difference shown in table III for serum calcium may perhaps be of clinical importance.

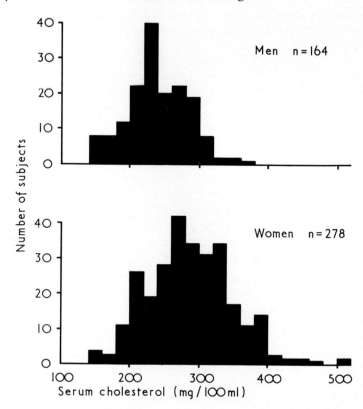

Frequency distribution of serum cholesterol in old people living at home.[18]

Phosphatases

It is uncertain whether the normal range of serum alkaline phosphatase is the same in young and old. A rise in mean values with age has long been attributed to an age-related increase in the prevalence of Paget's disease, and more recently to osteomalacia since the recognition that this disorder is common in elderly women.[32] Nevertheless, in elderly hospital patients, osteomalacia and Paget's disease are considerably less frequent conditions associated with a serum alkaline phosphatase above the conventional upper limit of normality of 15 King Armstrong units/100 ml than are liver disease, recent bone trauma, or malignant secondary deposits.[33] At present it would seem reasonable to regard a serum alkaline phosphatase of over 20 K-A units/100 ml as abnormal in an old person, and an indication for a search for liver or bone disease, and a value between 15 and 20 units as of uncertain significance. Values of over 50 units will usually be found to be due to Paget's disease, detectable either clinically or on a relatively restricted set of radiographs (for example, of the chest and pelvis), or to metastatic liver disease, of which there may be little other biochemical evidence. Determination of the iso-enzymes of alkaline phosphatase may be of great value, and wider availability of the test should help considerably in geriatric diagnosis.[34]

Normal values for the serum acid phosphatase are usually considered to be the same in the elderly as in middle age, and measurement of the tartrate-labile fraction (with due caution that a rectal examination has not recently been performed) is of great value in the diagnosis and management of prostatic carcinoma, one of the controllable cancers. There is nothing to suggest any age-related difference in the concentrations of other commonly estimated serum enzymes, such as aspartate transaminase, alanine transaminase, or lactic dehydrogenase.

TESTS OF ENDOCRINE FUNCTION

The endocrine disorders common in old age are diabetes mellitus. hyperthyroidism, and hypothyroidism. All others are distinctly rare, and only those tests relevant to the three common conditions mentioned will be discussed.

Diabetes

The most important single measurement in the diagnosis of diabetes is the random blood sugar. Values below 150 mg/100 ml may be accepted as normal in the elderly,[17] [35] and values over 200 mg/100 ml as indicative of diabetes—and thus requiring appropriate treatment. Most people with blood-sugar levels over 200 mg/100 ml have glycosuria, and many have frank diabetic symptoms—though these may only come to light on direct questioning. The difficulties concern those elderly people found to have random blood-sugar levels between 150 and 200 mg/100 ml. Consideration of all the circumstances, including the presence or absence of symptoms, repetition of the random blood sugar, or determination of the fasting blood sugar (a value of 130 mg/100 ml or more being taken to indicate diabetes) will help in deciding whether a diagnosis of diabetes is justified. Recourse to a glucose tolerance test may only increase the uncertainties, since many old people have tests in the "borderline" region, with a blood sugar two hours after glucose between 120 mg/100 ml—the level defining normality—and 200 mg/100 ml—the level defining diabetes.

Thyroid Disease

Of the numerous tests for thyroid function, those making use only of blood samples have much to recommend them in the diagnosis of thyroid disease in the elderly. The normal range of values of the serum protein-bound iodine (PBI) is usually taken to be the same in old age as earlier in life (that is, 4–9 µg/100 ml), but the assessment of values outside this range, both below and above, is often made difficult by several factors which are common in the elderly. Acutely ill elderly patients often have low values of PBI, owing to reduction in thyroxine-binding globulin levels.[36] Falsely high values are perhaps even more frequent, and result from iodine ingestion (particularly in cough medicines), and from a variety of drugs.[37] [38] A careful drug history is thus essential in assessing the significance of an abnormal PBI in an old person, but the use of the more recently introduced determinations of serum T-3 and T-4 levels is likely to be necessary to resolve many of these problems.[39] The greater availability of these tests will be of value in the diagnosis of these remediable disorders in old age.

CONCLUSION

Laboratory investigations are essential for the accurate diagnosis of many treatable conditions common in the elderly. The proper interpretation of the results of such investigations demands a knowledge both of the normal values encountered in old age and of the numerous factors which may produce misleading results.

REFERENCES

[1] Chalmers, D. G., Myers, A. M., and Saunders, C. R. G., Lancet, 1968, 2, 261.

[2] Nutritional Anaemias. W.H.O. Tech. Rep. Series No. 405, Geneva, 1968.

[3] Andrews, G. R., Caird, F. I., McLennan, W. J., and MacLeod, C., Quarterly Journal of Medicine, 1973, 42, 1.

[4] Powell, D. E. B. and Thomas, J. H., Blood Disorders in the Elderly, Wright, Bristol, 1971.

[5] Pirrie, R., Journal of Clinical Pathology, 1952, 5, 10.

[6] Bothwell, T. H., and Finch, C. A., Iron Metabolism, Little, Brown and Co., Boston, 1962.

[7] Bainton, D. F., and Finch, C. A., American Journal of Medicine, 1964, 37, 62.

[8] Mitchell, T. R., and Pegrum, G. D., Gerontologia Clinica, 1971, 13, 296.

[9] Dagg, J. H., Goldberg, A., MacFarlane, B., and Morrow, J. J., Quarterly Journal of Medicine, 1967, 36, 600.

[10] Dagg, J. H., Goldberg, A., and Morrow, J. J., Scottish Medical Journal, 1968, 13, 78.

[11] Elwood, P. C., and Hughes, D., British Medical Journal, 1970, 3, 254.

[12] Elwood, P. C., Hughes, D., Shinton, N. K., and Wrighton, R. J., British Medical Journal, 1970, 2, 458.

[13] Alexander, M. K., and Cruickshank, J. M., British Journal of Haematology, 1970, 18, 541.

[14] Andrews, G. R., Caird, F. I., and Gallie, T. B., Age and Ageing, 1972, 1, 239.

[15] Bottiger, L. E., and Svedberg, C. A., *British Medical Journal*, 1967, **2**, 85.

[16] Milne, J. S., and Williamson, J., *Gerontologia Clinica*, 1972, **14**, 36.

[17] Andrews, G. R., and Caird, F. I., Unpublished observations.

[18] Andrews, G. R., Caird, F. I., and Leask, R. G. S., *Age and Ageing*, 1973, **2**, 14.

[19] Judge, T. G., *Gerontologia Clinica*, 1968, **10**, 102.

[20] Shock, N. W., in *Surgery of the Aged and Debilitated Patient*, ed. J. H. Powers, p. 10. Philadelphia and London, Saunders, 1968.

[21] Campbell, H., Greene, W. J. W., Keyser, J. W., Waters, W. E. Weddell, J. M., and Withey, J. L., *British Journal of Preventive and Social Medicine*, 1968, **22**, 41.

[22] Grant, D. R., Kaufman, B. J., and Moorhouse, J. A., *Canadian Medical Association Journal*, 1969, **100**, 744.

Mental Disturbance in the Ill Old Person

BY

TOM DUNN, TOM ARIE

MENTAL disturbance is very common in ill old people and the mortality in this group is high. Management may be difficult and mismanagement can change a restless ill patient into an apathetic, dehydrated, incontinent patient with pressure sores, at grave risk of dying from pneumonia or pulmonary emboli.

Progressive mental impairment is a common accompaniment of ageing. Where this has progressed to obvious impairment of memory, the disability is labelled "dementia", but many of these old people (at least in the earlier years) remain sufficiently competent to go on living in a simpler way with their families or even by themselves. Even relatively mild physical illness or other adverse factors in such people can cause an acute confusional state, and precipitate a domestic crisis. Even when there is no obvious mental impairment the aged brain tends to have less "reserve", so that it is much more readily upset than the younger brain by drugs or illness. As a result over a third of all patients admitted directly to geriatric departments are confused.

The mental symptoms may range from delirium with hallucinations to restless, agitated, and aggressive behaviour. Many patients are obviously physically ill, but in some the psychiatric symptoms dominate the picture.

COMMONER CAUSES OF CONFUSIONAL STATES

Strokes

Patients with strokes causing major paralysis may be confused, but in these cases the cause is clear. Nevertheless, the cerebral infarction may not affect the pyramidal tracts, and the illness may then present with acute confusion. Careful examination may detect some confirmatory signs, such as minor weakness or clumsiness of a limb or an extensor plantar response. Examination must include rough tests of the visual fields, as homonymous hemianopia is easily missed in a confused person and it may contribute to the apparent confusion.

A stroke may cause only dysphasia, or even jargon aphasia, so that the patient's speech is gibberish. The patient may be confused or may only appear to be confused because of his nonsensical speech. Examination will reveal nominal dysphasia, and the sensible behaviour will be out of keeping with the disturbed speech. The disability can

78

be very frightening and bewildering to the patient, who may become agitated and frustrated—and this can add to the difficulty of diagnosis. At the onset of the stroke there may be headache, vomiting, vertigo, or ataxia as well as the acute onset of confusion. In many cases there will be no confirmatory signs and one is left with a presumptive diagnosis based on the history and on the exclusion of other factors. Electroencephalography may suggest focal damage, but whether further neurological investigation, including lumbar puncture, is justified depends on the history and total clinical picture. As with paralysis, there is a natural tendency for the confusional state to improve with time, though further strokes are common.

Cerebral Ischaemia

Many causes of cerebral ischaemia without actual infarction may cause confusion. A low cardiac output may be due to congestive heart failure, cardiac infarction, pulmonary emboli, or associated with abdominal emergencies such as volvulus, mesenteric infarction, or gastrointestinal bleeding. The patient is clearly ill, but the cause may not be obvious. Strokes and episodes of cerebral ischaemia are more common in patients with hypertension, but a normal or low blood pressure at the time of examination may be due to the ill state of the patient and evidence of previous hypertension may be found from left ventricular hypertrophy on x-ray examination and electrocardiography, or from examination of the optic fundi.

Cerebral Hypoxia

Patients with chronic respiratory failure readily become confused, especially with infection or with the onset of cor pulmonale, but may become lucid again as the acute episode subsides. Chronic anaemias cause confusion only when they are quite severe, with a haemoglobin level usually below 7 g/100 ml. Confusion may occur in vitamin B_{12} deficiency states, even without anaemia, but this responds to vitamin B_{12} injections only rarely.

Subdural Haematoma

This condition may be rewarding to find, and disastrous to miss. It must be suspected when there is a history of falls, and when confusion or consciousness is fluctuant. Old people with friable atheromatous vessels are particularly at risk, and there may be no clear history of trauma. Cortical atrophy seems also to predispose to collection of fluid in the laxer subdural space. Sometimes acute symptoms turn out to be associated with very old haematomas or hygromas, and even here the results of surgery may be excellent.

A prominent elderly local citizen had been noted to be progressively behaving more oddly over several months, a development which was attributed to his well-known fondness of alcohol. When he became acutely confused and agressive one Saturday night, the psychiatrist was summoned with a view to compulsory admission to hospital. In fact, he had papilloedema and minimal long-tract signs, and bilateral subdural hygromas of apparently very long standing were evacuated that night. He remained very confused for several weeks after operation but subsequently returned to full normality, with no detectable intellectual or neurological deficits, and was very well two years later.

Cerebral Tumour

A change in the behaviour and personality over a period of weeks or months may be the first evidence of cerebral tumour, either primary or secondary. When suspicion is aroused, either by the history or by the associated signs, full investigations will be required; often in this age group it is not reasonable to undertake operation, but in some patients, even the very old, surgery may be followed by worthwhile— and even dramatic—improvement.

Myxoedema

The mental symptoms of myxoedema are usually lethargy and slowing of thought processes. Occasionally there may be confusion, or a depressive or paranoid picture—the "myxoedematous madness" of Richard Asher. This may respond slowly to small doses of thyroxine; in most cases, however, the mental state is not improved, though the general physical state may be.

Diabetes

Diabetic hyperglycaemia or acidosis may present with confusion as well as drowsiness. More frequent, and much more important, is the confusional state due to hypoglycaemia, especially from oral antidiabetic drugs. Diabetes is common in old people and many are unnecessarily started on oral drugs when the mild diabetes could be controlled by diet only. The hypoglycaemia may be far from obvious as it often presents as a confusional state without sweating or hypotension. It may come on insidiously and persist for hours or even for days if the treatment is continued. It should always be suspected when there is confused behaviour of someone on oral hypoglycaemic drugs. If confirmation from blood sugar estimation (or Dextrostix) is not readily available, it may be obtained by the therapeutic response to a large dose (for example, 25 g) of intravenous glucose or to oral carbohydrate. Chlorpropamide is not the drug of first choice in the elderly because its long action makes hypoglycaemia particularly dangerous. A diguanide such as phenformin may be sufficient but if a sulphonylurea is required one of the shorter acting drugs such as tolbutamide is safer. Chronic brain failure is common in diabetes, probably because of increased prevalence of atheroma, but sometimes because of past cerebral damage from severe hypoglycaemia.

Toxic Causes

Infections

In a young person high fever or pneumonia may cause delirium, but in older people delirium may accompany less severe infections. In old people infections—for example, pneumonia or urinary infections— may be silent till they are quite advanced and a change in the mental state is often the presenting symptom.

Tissue Necrosis

The mental state of a patient ill and confused with gangrene of a leg may be much improved after amputation. In the same way a major pressure sore may contribute to the confusion of the patient already ill enough to develop a sore. Absorption of blood, either from a large haematoma (which may accompany a fracture of the femur) or from the gut after gastrointestinal haemorrhage, may exacerbate both the physical and the mental state.

Other Toxic Causes

Chronic renal failure is common and with the associated anaemia can make the patient ill and confused; it may also add to the illness by enhancing the toxicity of drugs. Pre-renal uraemia may result from an inadequate fluid intake. Electrolyte imbalance may be due to dehydration, renal failure, or to drugs, or to a combination of these factors.

Carcinoma without cerebral metastases may affect the nervous system by causing toxic neuropathy or occasionally cerebellar-degeneration; it may also cause or exacerbate confusion.

Drugs

Old people tend to have multiple diseases, and it is all too easy to give a drug for each condition that one finds—for hypertension, methyldopa; for giddiness, prochlorperazine; for ankle oedema, irrespective of cause, a diuretic; for anxiety, a tranquillizer; and so on.

Old people's brains are quite easily befuddled and they are often subjected to greater concentrations of drugs than those of the young, partly because of the number of drugs prescribed, partly because a

F

degree of renal failure impairs excretion, and partly because so often a frail old lady has such a small body mass. It is important to avoid overtreating elderly people. Time after time we have seen a remarkable improvement in the physical and mental state when all the numerous drugs have been stopped. If the elderly patient is on a complicated regimen it is virtually certain that the regimen will not be properly followed, and it may be the important drugs which are omitted. This is likely to make evaluation even more difficult, because one can never be certain what the patient is actually taking. It should seldom be necessary to prescribe more than three different regular drugs. When a drug is prescribed, it should be discontinued when it is no longer needed.

The drugs which are mostly likely to cause confusion are those which are directly on the nervous system—and the most notorious are the anti-Parkinsonian drugs.

A patient was admitted in a confused agitated state, tottery and having had some falls. Over the next day or two he returned to his normal slightly forgetful self and after returning home to his elderly wife he remained well for a week. He then again became acutely confused and that night fell on getting out of bed and was incontinent of faeces. This crisis precipitated a home visit next day, when a bottle of benzhexol tablets were found. Inquiry showed that they had been started just before the first admission, but had not been resumed after discharge till the previous day when his wife asked the district nurse if she should restart them. One tablet was apparently enough to cause this crisis.

All the anticholinergic drugs as well as L-dopa and amantadine may cause insomnia, restlessness, hallucinations, and delusions. The inital doses of these drugs must be small and the level built up gradually; only rarely should they be pressed to the levels used in younger people.

All sedatives and tranquillizers are apt to make an ill old person bemused and lethargic and add to the difficulties of nursing care. They can also cause hypotension with fainting or falls and can contribute to hypothermia. They may be necessary to control restlessness or delusions, but when they must be prescribed the starting dose should be less than in younger people. Hypnotics too increase the liability to falls during the night and may cause nocturnal confusion. It is hardly ever necessary for old people to have hypnotics regularly. When prescribed for a single occasion or for a short spell the dose should be lower than in younger people whatever hypnotic is used.

Tricyclic antidepressants are valuable, but may cause excitement and confusion. Monoamine-oxidase inhibitors are only very rarely appropriate for old people, and it is obviously of particular importance to satisfy oneself that the patient or her attendants can be relied upon to keep to the necessary dietary restriction. Finally, the doctor must not forget that elderly people as well as younger people may be alcoholics, with ataxia and a chronic befuddled state.

Epilepsy

Epilepsy is common in older people and is most commonly due to arteriosclerotic brain damage. The seizures may be followed by a period of drowsy confusion, but are often atypical and may present as transient episodes of confused behaviour. In the elderly the doses of antiepileptic drugs used in younger people often cause unsteadiness and confusion.

Multiple Factors

Often it is not possible to point to a single cause of confusion in an ill old person. It may be due partly to the primary illness, partly to removal from familiar surroundings, partly to dehydration or electrolyte disturbance, partly to the complications of venous thrombosis or pressure sores, and partly to the drugs used. If there is any underlying dementia then the more severe the dementia the less specific and clear-cut the cause of a confusional state is likely to be.

PRINCIPLES OF DIAGNOSIS AND MANAGEMENT

Diagnosis

It is important to obtain a full history of the development of the illness and this must include a history from a relative, friend, or neighbour. It is very important to ascertain the mental state of the patient *before* the illness. The abrupt onset of confusion suggests the possibility of a stroke. The development of confused behaviour over some weeks or months in a previously normal person raises the possibility of a cerebral tumour. A history of previous mental illness—for example, depression— even many years ago, may be a valuable clue.

An 82-year-old woman, evidently very confused, but talking very little, incontinent and refusing food and drink, was admitted to our joint unit. The recent history was not clear, but a relatively sudden deterioration seemed to have occurred. The family said there was no previous history of psychiatric illness. The lady looked sad, and the nursing staff were asked to keep a careful record of the few utterances she made. Such as there were turned out to be almost all self-depreciating, and a diagnosis of depression was made. Despite general measures she continued to decline, and she was given electroplexy to which she made a gratifying response. It was only at this point that the family "confessed" that she had had an almost identical illness 20 years ago, when she had likewise recovered after electroplexy.

The inquiry must include a drug history and especially the relation of the onset of confusion to any new therapy. Physical examination may be difficult, but must not be neglected, and should include neurological examination.

The cause of the illness and the mental disturbance will often then be clear and, if the facilities are adequate, the patient can be managed at home. When the cause is not clear, the advice of a geriatric physician or psychiatrist should be sought at a domiciliary consultation. When the cause cannot be established at home, or when sufficient facilities, or tolerance, to nurse the patient at home are not readily available, the patient must be admitted to hospital. Because the accent will normally be on physical investigations and general nursing care, admission should be sought not to a psychiatric department, but to the geriatric or medical department. Where there is a "psychogeriatric assessment unit" jointly controlled by a psychiatrist and the geriatrician, admission to this unit may be best.

Management

The management of an ill confused old person is one of the most difficult problems in the practice of medicine. Every effort must be made to find and treat the underlying cause or causes, not just to treat the mental disturbance symptomatically. While waiting for treatment to take effect or for natural recovery, symptomatic and supportive treatment will be necessary.

If the patient is restless, sedation will probably be required—but strong sedation is likely to add to the gravity of the primary illness. If the patient is ambulant, sedation will make him liable to fall. If sedation is sufficient to keep him in bed, it is likely to lead to pressure sores, venous thrombosis, or serious dehydration. Even without sedation it may be difficult to get adequate fluids into ill confused patients (a careful record should always be kept of fluid intake and, so far as possible, of output).

For these reasons the least possible sedation should be used. The more nursing time that can be devoted to the patient the less will be the need for sedatives and the easier it will be to maintain an adequate fluid intake. Where there is a willing relative this will be best achieved at home; moreover, the patient may be less disorientated in his own surroundings and with his own family. Reassurance, familiar attendants, and, in hospital, minimum change of surroundings are all as important as sedative drugs. Good lighting can be important; some patients become much more confused in shadowy ill-lit rooms. Disturbed behaviour is apt to be worse at night and more distressing to relatives, who themselves become irritable through lack of sleep; so hypnotics will usually be required. The most popular hypnotics in geriatric practice are those short-acting drugs based on chloral hydrate, or one 5 mg tablet of nitrazepam. When there is restlessness, however, a phenothiazine will be indicated—for example, chlorpromazine 25 mg or thioridazine, which may be given together with a mild hypnotic drug. When restlessness is a problem by day, regular rather than sporadic phenothiazine drugs are usually best. In old and frail people we prefer promazine, say 25 mg three times a day, rather than stronger phenothiazines, because the dose of the weaker drug may be more exactly adjusted. Such drugs are cumulative and the effect increases over the first day or two. There is much to be said for the doctor relying on one or two major tranquillizers with which he is familiar, rather than trying out the latest one. Long-acting injected tranquillizers such as fluphenazine decanoate are best avoided in old people, because, once injected, their dosage cannot be regulated and side effects may be very troublesome. When the patient cannot be controlled by these means, or when dehydration threatens to become a problem, admission to hospital will be indicated. It may then be necessary to rehydrate the patient, by giving heavy sedation so that he will not interfere with a stomach tube or intravenous infusions. A wild and aggressive patient who cannot be calmed may need more dramatic action. Chlorpromazine, 50 mg by injection, will usually be effective, but this should be a single dose and not repeated regularly without reassessment.

We know of no good evidence that it helps to give massive doses of vitamins to confused patients. It is reasonable to give vitamins in therapeutic doses to those patients who have been living in a state of neglect and malnutrition, and, of course, especially if alcoholism is known or suspected. Search for bottles should be part of the routine assessment of the elderly recluse or isolate.

DEPRESSION

Depression in old people may respond excellently to drug treatment or to electroplexy and it may present as a confusional state. The past history is a particularly important feature. The patient may be agitated, but more often is withdrawn or even mute, refusing food and drink, so that she becomes dehydrated and seriously ill. Confirmation of the diagnosis should be sought from a psychiatrist. Admission will be required for the more severe cases either to a psychiatric department or to a joint geriatric-psychiatric unit.

A 68-year-old man "collapsed" while visiting his wife, who had for many years been a patient in a mental hospital. He was himself admitted to hospital, but despite extensive investigations no physical cause for his "collapse" was found; but he was confused, withdrawn, refused food, and looked sad. It turned out that his dog, with whom he had lived alone for many years since his wife's hospitalization, had recently died, and his neighbours had noticed that he had virtually stopped going out. A diagnosis of depression was made, though some degree of dementia was also suspected. Treatment with amitriptyline was started but he become still further dehydrated and was transferred to a geriatric unit. He became grossly confused, withdrawn, and ill. He was rehydrated, an intercurrent chest infection was treated, and he was given electroplexy, whereupon he recovered to full normality with no signs of intellectual impairment. Six months later he wrote a long and impeccable letter reporting his progress, having moved to another part of the country, to which he wished also to bring his wife.

DELUSIONAL STATES

Chronic delusional states without progressive dementia, usually paranoid, are common in old people. They can often live with their delusions quite happily, though they may cause concern to others. With new physical illness the delusional state may become more severe or come to the notice of the doctor for the first time. Their persecutory states often respond to phenothiazine treatment, sometimes dramatically.

Skeletal Disease in the Elderly

BY

JAMES T. LEEMING

MUCH useful research is being carried out on bone disorders and bone physiology at present and our understanding of the relevant metabolic processes is expanding rapidly. Though this increased knowledge has greatly increased our awareness of the aetiological and therapeutic possibilities, in general it has not yet had a great impact on routine diagnosis and treatment. Two examples of these advances are worth citing—namely, the discovery of the hormone calcitonin, produced in the thyroid gland, and the advances in knowledge concerning vitamin D metabolism.

Calcitonin inhibits bone resorption and thus counterbalances the effect of parathyroid hormone. Other substances, such as glucagon and gastrin stimulate the release of calcitonin. It is not yet known, however, how important these interrelationships are in the average person—whether reduced production of calcitonin is a major factor in producing osteoporosis, or whether established oesteoporosis can be effectively treated with it.

Advances in knowledge of vitamin D metabolism have been equally impressive. Vitamin D_3 (cholecalciferol) is now known to be converted in the liver to another substance (25-hydroxy-D_3) and the kidneys then convert it yet again into two further compounds (1, 25-dihydroxy-D_3, and 21, 25-dihydroxy-D_3), the first of which acts on bone more quickly than the second. These discoveries open up immense new possibilities regarding the pathogenesis and treatment of vitamin D deficiency, but it is too early yet for them to affect routine clinical practice.

PRACTICAL ASPECTS

The remainder of this article will concentrate on practical aspects of bone disorders as they present in the elderly. In general, patients over 75 will be under consideration, though in calculating prevalence it is convenient to use the age of 65. Mention will be made of four conditions: (1) osteoporosis; (2) Paget's disease; (3) osteomalacia; and (4) malignant disease, including multiple myeloma.

It is important to consider the frequency with which these conditions are likely to occur in an average practice. A general practitioner's list of 3,000 patients will be assumed to have 360 patients over the age of 65 (220 women and 140 men). A geriatric department serving a population of 240,000 and admitting 1,000 patients a year will be assumed to serve 80 general practitioners.

Osteoporosis, with a liability to fracture, affects 25% of women over the age of 65, and men are probably affected a quarter as frequently as women. The incidence of Paget's disease rises to 10% by the age of 90, so an incidence of 6% will be assumed for those over 65. Men are affected more often than women. Osteomalacia, mostly occurring in women, is found in between 1 and 4% of geriatric hospital admissions (the higher figure in Glasgow and the lower figure in the south of England).

By using these figures and assumptions it will be expected that a general practitioner with a list of 3,000 will have on his list 70 patients with osteoporosis (55 women and 9 men), 20 patients with Paget's disease (about 12 men and 8 women), and that he will see a case of osteomalacia once every two to eight years. The incidence of malignant disease of bone has not been calculated but will not be high.

In the table the incidence of these conditions is compared and they are placed very broadly in order with regard to preventability, treatability, and seriousness if untreated.

Incidence	Preventability
Osteoporosis+ + + Paget's+ + Osteomalacia± Malignancy±	Osteomalacia+ + + Osteoporosis± Paget's O Malignancy O

Treatability	Seriousness if not Treated
Osteomalacia+ + + Paget's+ + Malignancy+ Osteoporosis±	Malignancy+ + + Osteomalacia+ + Osteoporosis+ Paget's±

O — + + + = rough guide to importance of each disease under each heading.

The less common conditions merit more emphasis than their incidence would suggest because they can be treated and cause more trouble if untreated; osteomalacia can be prevented and so may osteoporosis in a more limited sense. All four conditions lead to bones being fractured by relatively minor trauma so that this is not a useful way of differentiating them. The fact that fractures may easily occur in the elderly should constantly be borne in mind, however, because the absence of severe trauma and the presence of other diseases make it easy to overlook them. Thus the patient with a hemiplegia may have a fractured neck of femur on the same side, the lady with painful arthritis of the hips may fracture the neck of the femur, and the patient with cracked and painful ribs due to osteomalacia may also have angina and may be too anxious or confused to give a clear description.

OSTEOPOROSIS

Osteoporosis signifies a generalized loss of bone, the bone which remains being normal. The serum calcium, phosphorus, and alkaline phosphatase levels are not affected and there are no symptoms or signs till structural failure occurs. Recent work has established that the amount of bone in the skeleton increases till the age of 20–25, after which it very slowly declines. Women accumulate less bone than men and tend to lose it more quickly. Structural failure usually begins in women over the age of 50 and in men over the age of about 65. It shows itself in a loss of height and thoracic kyphosis due to narrowing of the vertebral bodies and a wedge-shaped deformity of the thoracic vertebrae. The lower ribs sink towards the iliac crest. The clinical features have been reviewed by Dent and Watson.[1] Fractures occur in the lower forearm in women over the age of 50 and in the neck of the femur in both sexes over the age of 70. Compression fractures occur from time to time in the lower thoracic and lumbar vertebrae, which characteristically produce severe localized backache which clears up in three to four weeks. Neurological sequelae rarely if ever occur. Probably vertebral fractures are often not recognized at the time. Recognition is made more difficult by the fact that only a minority of cases of backache can be traced to osteoporosis.[2]

Though osteoporosis is, broadly speaking, a benign condition, it exacts a considerable price in terms of episodic morbidity, the consequences becoming more serious with increasing age. Treatment has so far been able only to arrest the condition rather than cure it. It is possible, but not certain, that a little fluoride in the drinking water in early life may lead to the production of a better skeleton. Oestrogens have been said to prevent parathyroid-mediated bone resorption, and minor degrees of vitamin D deficiency may also have aetiological relevance. Larger doses of fluoride have been used in therapy. There is considerable debate, however, about the value of these agents in treatment and the main emphasis should be on minimizing the two factors most certain to increase osteoporosis—namely, bed rest and steroid therapy. It is in this sense that osteoporosis may be called preventable. Bed rest has repeatedly been shown to lead to a negative calcium balance.[3] Hypercalciuria persists even if the legs are exercised in bed.

To prevent excessive bone loss, therefore, periods of bed rest should be kept as short as possible throughout life. The administration of adrenocortical steroids also has a powerful effect in increasing osteoporosis[4] and this should not be overlooked when they are prescribed. When fractures occur they should be treated promptly and analgesics prescribed to permit a speedy return to normal activity. Temporary admission to hospital may be indicated to achieve quicker mobilization. Attention to the other medical and social conditions so often present in old people will help to increase mobility and also reduce the likelihood of falls in the future. Home conditions should be investigated and hazards removed or alleviated wherever possible. Diet should be adequate and varied, especially with regard to calcium and vitamin D. A daily pint of milk is the best source of calcium.

PAGET'S DISEASE

Paget's disease affects the skeleton in a patchy, asymmetrical manner and is not generalized. Most commonly affected are the pelvis, lumbar spine, femur, tibia, skull, and clavicle. At the affected sites there is a greatly increased bone turnover. The new bone is spongy and disorganized. Expansion and deformity occur in affected bones and gross bowing may occur in the femur and tibia. It is a disease which may have phases of activity and inactivity. During active phases the affected bone is warm to the touch and the serum alkaline phosphatase level may be grossly raised. The serum calcium and phosphorus levels are usually normal. The increased circulation through the affected bone may sometimes precipitate or exacerbate heart failure but this seems to happen very little in the elderly. Pain in the affected bone may be severe, but this also is uncommon in my experience. Common practical problems stem from gross deformities and from nerve deafness due to compression of the 8th nerve by the enlarged bone. Paget's disease varies enormously in extent, sometimes only one clavicle being affected. In rare instances when the spine is affected neurological effects such as paraplegia may be produced.

Apart from simple symptomatic measures treatment is rarely necessary in Paget's disease, but recently, calcitonin (give by injection once or twice daily) has been found to be effective. It has produced relief from pain, a fall in the serum alkaline phosphatase level, and improvement in the bony appearances. It use should be considered when pain is severe and prolonged or if there is reason to expect serious complications, such as paraplegia.

OSTEOMALACIA

Osteomalacia is characterized histologically by failure of newly formed bone (osteoid) to calcify. The serum calcium and phosphorus levels are often, though not invariably, reduced and the serum alkaline phosphatase level is raised in 80% of cases. Iliac crest bone biopsy, which can be performed using a local anaesthetic, is the most reliable single method of diagnosis.

Weakness of the proximal limb muscles is a major manifestation and leads to difficulty lifting the feet over kerbstones and ultimately to the necessity of going up and downstairs on all fours. The gait may be rolling or "waddling" in character. This weakness can often be shown by formal neurological examination in young subjects, but in old patients the presence of multiple pathology usually prevents a convincing display. Difficulty in walking or an inability to walk is a leading symptom, however, and myopathy can be inferred from this. Bone pain—especially in the back, thighs, shoulder region, or ribs is usually present—and the bones may be tender. The pain is worse on muscular effort. Quite often, especially in those patients seen in geriatric departments, the pain is vague and undramatic. Characteristically it occurs in several of the above sites. Fractures of the ribs are more common in osteomalacia than in osteoporosis, and possibly their significance has sometimes been underestimated. The clinical features were reviewed by Chalmers.[5]

Osteomalacia is more common after partial gastrectomy, in patients on phenobarbitone and other anticonvulsants, and when there is intestinal malabsorption. Until recently is was thought that the commonest cause in old age was inadequate diet, but recently lack of sunshine has been thought especially important.[6] The disorder occurs more often in the housebound.[7] When venous blood is taken to support the diagnosis the patients should be fasting and it is important to use only the minimum tourniquet pressure. The serum proteins and blood urea should be estimated at the same time because a reduction of the albumin level will lead to a lowering of serum calcium and a raised urea will cause a rise in the serum phosphorus. It is worth checking the blood count at the same time to exclude anaemia. X-ray films of the chest, lumbar spine, and pelvis are helpful, partly to exclude Paget's disease as the cause for a raised serum alkaline phosphatase and partly because the presence of incomplete fractures (Looser's zones) in the pubic rami, femoral neck, axillary border of scapula, or upper end of the humerus is virtual proof of the diagnosis. Unfortunately they are only seen in a minority of cases.

As it is curable, osteomalacia should be excluded in any old person who is bedfast or having difficulty getting about without obvious cause, or when the above symptoms are present. Bone biospy should be done in doubtful cases and is frequently advisable.

Hence osteomalacia is a difficult condition to diagnose in hospital without bone biopsy. It is even more difficult in general practice, where it occurs much less frequently. The best plan, therefore, is to refer suspected patients to hospital for further investigation. Once diagnosed the condition is not difficult to treat. A suggested scheme is to give calciferol 50,000 units (1·25 mg) daily for two weeks followed by tablets of calcium and vitamin D (*BPC*) in a dose of one tablet twice daily for 12 months. It is important not to prolong treatment with the larger dose of calciferol, which would be liable to produce hypercalcaemia followed by renal failure.

Bone pain usually clears and the serum calcium and phosphorus return to normal within two weeks, but it may be six to eight months before the serum alkaline phosphatase level falls to within normal limits. When treatment is begun the serum alkaline phosphatase level often rises temporarily.

Regular Prophylaxis

To prevent a recurrence of osteomalacia and to prevent its development in housebound patients over the age of 75, it is logical to give regular prophylactic vitamin D, such as Tabs calcium with vitamin D (*BPC*), which contain 500 units of vitamin D, or vitamin A and D capsules (*BPC*), which contain 450 units, in a dose of one tablet or capsule daily for three or four months during the winter. Even small amounts of exposure to the sun are beneficial and should be encouraged.

It is worth noting that osteomalacia may occur in patients with other more obvious bone disorders. Thus I have seen bone pain in a patient with breast metastases and backache in a patient with Paget's disease clear up when vitamin D was given. The serum phosphorus level was initially low in both patients. A therapeutic trial of vitamin D (for example, 50,000 units daily for not more than a week or two) is well justified in this situation.

MALIGNANT DISEASE

Multiple myeloma is not rare in hospital practice. It causes bone pain often in several sites and a liability to pathological fractures. The serum calcium level may be normal or raised, the serum phosphorus and alkaline phosphatase concentrations are normal. X-ray films show clear-cut translucencies which are especially easy to recognize in a lateral view of the skull. Anaemia and renal failure may be complications and Bence-Jones protein may be found in the urine. The erythrocyte sedimentation rate is usually high and the serum globulin level considerably raised.

With modern methods of treatment including radiotherapy, melphalan, cyclophosphamide, and steroids (often in combination and given intermittently) much can be done to relieve symptoms and prolong life, and multiple myeloma should no longer be dismissed as untreatable.

Bony metastases from carcinoma of the prostrate and carcinoma of the breast may cause much pain and disability. They are usually fairly simple to spot in x-ray films. They cause a rise of the serum alkaline phosphatase level and sometimes also of the serum calcium. If carcinoma of the prostate is the cause there is usually a rise of the serum acid phosphatase level. Considerable relief may be produced by appropriate drugs such as oestrogens and steroids for breast cancer metastases and oestrogens for prostatic cancer metastases.

REFERENCES

[1] Dent, C. E., and Watson, L., *Postgraduate Medical Journal*, 1966, **42**, 581.
[2] Adams, P., Davies, G. T., and Sweetnam, P., *Quarterly Journal of Medicine*, 1970, **39**, 601.
[3] Moore Ede, M. C., Faulkner, M. H., and Tredre, B. E., *Clinical Science*, 1972, **42**, 433.
[4] Cope, C. L., in *Adrenal Steroids and Disease*, 2nd edition, p. 535. Pitman Medical, London, 1972.
[5] Chalmers, J., *Journal of the Royal College of Physicians of Edinburgh*, 1968, **13**, 255.
[6] Hodkinson, H. M., Stanton, B. R., Round, P., and Morgan, C., *Lancet*, 1973, **1**, 910.
[7] Leeming, J. T., Webster, S. G. P., Whitaker, R. S., and Wilkinson, M., Communication to British Geriatrics Society, April, 1973.

The following leading articles discuss the subjects indicated:
(1) Calcitonin and metabolic bone disease: *Lancet*, 1971, **1**, 1168.
(2) New ideas on Vitamin D: *British Medical Journal*, 1973, **1**, 629.
(3) Osteoporosis: *British Medical Journal*, 1971, **1**, 566.
(4) Fluoride and osteoporosis: *British Medical Journal*, 1972, **4**, 748.
(5) Treatment of Paget's disease of bone: *Lancet*, 1973, **1**, 1043.
(6) Compression of cord by Paget's disease: *British Medical Journal*, 1973, **2**, 321.
(7) The need for vitamin D supplements: *Lancet*, 1973, **1**, 1097.

Dementia in the Elderly: Diagnosis and Assessment

BY

TOM ARIE

FEW patients are so taxing to doctors as the confused and demented. No other condition generates so much crisis, irritability, and inter-professional friction. Dementia is common: about 10% of old people are demented, half of them severely, and in the over-80s this proportion rises to more than one in five. Most are women, because among the very old women outnumber men by over two to one. There will be even more old people with dementia as the number of old people, and particularly the very old, continues to increase.

Until recently virtually no doctors took any interest in dementia, with a few outstanding exceptions. Yet an average general practitioner's list is likely to contain about 30–40 demented patients, and every general practitioner knows that the demands that many of these patients will make are out of proportion to their numbers, not least because their problems often present as crises.

It is not difficult to see why the "psychogeriatric crisis" is so common; one reason is that dementia heads the list of important conditions among elderly patients at home of which their general practitioners are likely to be unaware. Williamson and his colleagues in Edinburgh found that over 80% of moderately or severely demented old people were not known to be so to their general practitioners. Since these patients only very rarely seek medical help for themselves, not surprisingly they produce crises when their disabilities impinge on others or are "unmasked" by the death of a spouse, or the marriage of a daughter. Preventive measures must be based on the general-practice team, but the high rate of admission of old people to hospital means that every admission gives an important opportunity for screening the patient's mental function.

WHAT IS DEMENTIA?

Dementia in the elderly is a global disruption of personality, affecting behaviour and intelligence, with impairment of the ability to learn new responses—and thus to adapt to a changing environment. The emotional response is disorganized and blunted, and, most striking of all, there is loss of the ability to remember recent events. Often an astonishing degree of function may be preserved, provided

94

the old person retains a constant environment with which she is familiar and that new demands on her are not great. Even so, such preservation is always precarious, depending on a constancy and security which are unlikely to last for long.

Senile and Arteriosclerotic Dementia

Dementia is of two main types, senile and arteriosclerotic. In the former there is degeneration of the parenchymatous tissue of the brain, the rate of which is mainly determined genetically. In the latter the brain substance degenerates as the result of impaired blood supply, with disseminated softenings due to infarction. In senile dementia the surface of the brain shrinks, the sulci are widened, and the ventricles dilated; most commonly, the parietal lobes are particularly affected. The pathological process in senile dementia is the same as that in Alzheimer's presenile dementia, the difference between "presenile" and "senile" Alzheimer's dementia being the genetically determined early onset and more rapid progression of the former. Other rare types of presenile dementia include Pick's disease (affecting chiefly the frontal lobes), Jakob-Creutzfeldt disease (which usually runs a very rapid course), and Huntington's chorea (with an autosomal dominant inheritance, the gross clinical manifestations of which are only very rarely delayed until late life).

By contrast, in arteriosclerotic dementia the deficits are attributable to the site of vascular damage; thus a patient may have much brain damage without dementia, but dementia is unlikely to occur without a certain minimum volume of brain having been destroyed. Whereas senile dementia generally follows a steady downhill course, a "step-wise" course is typical in arteriosclerotic dementia, often with relatively lucid intervals. During these intervals the patient may retain so much insight into his own predicament that his plight is one of the most pitiful in medicine. There is often a shallow lability of mood, in which the patient is laughing at one moment and crying the next, and this makes it easy to miss the depressive state which is common in these patients, which often responds well to antidepressant drugs or electroplexy. A history of hypertension and strokes is common. Epilepsy is much more common in arteriosclerotic than in senile dementia.

Some patients have both senile and arteriosclerotic brain damage simultaneously, since both are common. Wandering, incontinence, and impaired capacity for self-care are features of both conditions, as are paranoid developments; visual hallucinations are more characteristic of arteriosclerotic dementia. Neuropathological studies have confirmed that clinical distinction between the two types of dementia is fairly accurate, and there is a relationship between the characteristic histological changes in the brain in senile dementia ("senile plaques" and neurofibrillary tangles) and its clinical severity. The expectation of life for both groups is from a quarter to a half that normal for the age.

Other Causes of Dementia

Other causes of dementia are listed for completeness, but in the absence of specific evidence most of them are uncommon. They are: tumours, subdural haematomas, giant aneurysms; trauma, including the chronic trauma of boxers; syphilis and non-syphilitic inflammatory disease; chronic alcoholism; "normal pressure" or "communicating" hydrocephalus; myxoedema; vitamin B_{12} deficiency; chronic epilepsy; carcinomatosis.

Amnestic States

In amnestic states, the commonest of which is Korsakoff's psychosis of chronic alcoholics, there is a specific defect of recent memory, without the damage to personality, intelligence, and emotion. The sparing of intelligence is shown by the ingenuity of the "confabulation" which fills the deficit of memory. The syndrome may present acutely or subacutely as a confusional state, with the ataxia, eye-signs (most commonly nystagmus), and peripheral neuritis of Wernicke's encephalopathy. The neurological features of thiamine deficiency almost always respond quite rapidly to parenteral vitamins in high dosage, but the mental changes improve more slowly and not always completely.

Acute Confusional States

Almost any physical, social, or psychological disturbance in an old person may produce a confusional state (acute delirium). In arteriosclerotic dementia such acute episodes are common, but in general, the more severe the underlying dementia, the more readily may an acute confusional episode be precipitated; and, the more demented the patient, the less specific may be the precipitants of the confusional state.

WHY DOES DEMENTIA SO OFTEN PRESENT AS A CRISIS?

Obviously an old person who is demented but not known to be so is more likely suddenly to catch the doctor unawares than is one for whom measures of support have already been brought to bear. Crises are inconvenient, unpleasant, and difficult to deal with coolly—for anxiety is readily communicable. Crises are inherent in this work, and they cannot be wholly "organised away"; but insight into their genesis should help to make them more intelligible, less common, and perhaps even more bearable. The following rough classification is suggested.

Firstly, something has happened to the patient, such as a development in the dementing process—for instance, in the case of arteriosclerotic dementia, a stroke or an intercurrent illness. Often such a change will present as acute confusion.

Secondly, something has happened in the environment, such as a sudden change in support—for instance, the main caring relative has been admitted to hospital, or has died; or a patient who lives alone has suddenly been discharged from hospital, with no evident forethought about her capacity to cope. Often the event is less straightforward: tolerance of the old person may snap because of a marital row in the family caring for her, or the family may become anxious about the effect of the confused old lady on a teenager who is working for exams.

Thirdly, "enough is enough": people can take so much, and then often no more, particularly when no end is in sight. Thus the old lady may wander out of her house in her underclothes and be cheerfully fielded back, but when she has done so a second or third, or a tenth time, tolerance may break—especially if the caring service has not responded adequately.

Fourthly, the crisis may be a manipulation of the caring system, for one or more of the following reasons.

Poor Local Services

If it is impossible, or thought to be impossible, to get help from local services in response to cool and reasoned referral, then families and general practitioners will understandably have recourse to declaring an emergency. It follows that where a well-run service is established there is invariably a fall in the rate of crisis referrals (and an increase in referrals as a whole).

Ignorance

Many doctors and social workers cannot formulate a "psycho-geriatric" problem in any other terms but as the need to get it instantly off their hands. They are most unlikely ever to have had training in these matters—a state of affairs which is slowly improving for doctors, and rapidly deteriorating for social workers. A subcategory of this group are those who become irritable and resentful when asked to deal with anything but a straightforward somatic problem: these are the "limited graduates" described by Walton and his colleagues.[1]

Guilt

A common manifestation is the "Monday morning syndrome" familiar to many general practitioners, psychiatrists, geriatricians, and their secretaries. An old lady, often doing quite well, if not perfectly well, is living on her own and her children come for their quarterly

Sunday visit. They see she could well do with rather more care than she is having, but are unable or unwilling to provide it themselves. They telephone the general practitioner "first thing on Monday morning" to say that "something must be done".

The "Preventive Crisis"

This paradoxically is an example of forethought, though this is rarely carried over into the general management. We call it the "Friday afternoon crisis", and it derives from the fact that those concerned with the patient—relatives or professional attendants—are planning to go away for the weekend.

This list oversimplifies: the genesis of crises is always multifactorial.

ASSESSMENT

An organic psychiatric syndrome should always be assessed initially at home because it is an old person's capacity to function in her normal surroundings that needs to be assessed. Assessment at home also makes it possible to see the physical surroundings and often to make practical suggestions for domestic rearrangements. Members of the family and neighbours should be interviewed—and one cannot overstress that a reliable history obtained from others is paramount in assessing dementia. It will often be helpful for a social worker to be present, so that discussion and joint decisions can take place on the spot; alternatively, the health visitor or the district nurse may be the most appropriate colleague to accompany the general practitioner.

It is always wise to inquire whether the patient is already known to the social services department, since general practitioners are not always notified when confused old people are referred direct to the social services by relatives or neighbours. If after initial assessment specialist help seems to be needed then it will usually be best for the specialist also to see the patient at home.

Only rarely can general practitioner, social worker, and specialist all visit at the same time (as the Government circular on *Psycho-Geriatric Assessment Units* suggests); it is more important that they should be easily accessible and able to discuss a case together.

The History

The assessment begins with a history from a relative, neighbour, or other informant. I prefer to obtain this initial history before I meet the patient, who is often in another room and unaware of one's arrival. Once one becomes engaged with a demented person it is often very difficult to disengage again—if one excuses oneself to go and talk to a relative, the patient is likely to become anxious, wondering what one is up to, and to interrupt with repetitive perseverating, questioning, repeatedly coming back into the room. The history from the relative usually helps to orient oneself to the problem so that the subsequent interviews with the patient may be better directed to the points at issue.

Examination

The assessment itself follows general principles of physical and mental examination. Some points should be noted routinely, as follows.

General Appearance

Is the patient's general appearance compatible with the history?
Do the mental and physical states more or less match each other?
Are any of the following present: anaemia, myxoedema, or neurological and locomotor deficits?
Is the patient deaf (using a deaf aid?) or blind?
Is there chestiness or heart failure?
Is she smelly or wet?

State of the Household

If the old person lives alone, the state of her home will often be the best measure of her capacity for self-care (though one must take care to establish what help she is having from others). The kitchen and the contents of the larder are particular eloquent—what was the last meal, how much of it has been eaten, is there any accumulation of bottles? More generally, is the place clean, is it warm; is there gross neglect of hygiene; signs that the bed has been slept in?

Mental Examination

The mental examination follows standard lines, but is particularly directed to assessment of cognitive functions, largely by finding out the patient's grasp of the material of everyday life. The examination must be unhurried, and the patient will need a few moments to take in what is happening. A strange man suddenly appearing off the street and immediately asking "What is the name of the Prime Minister?" is likely either to put the final touch to the patient's confusion, or to convince her that she has fallen into the hands of a madman. One should explain carefully who one is (I usually also ask the patient to remember my name, which I then repeat to her, explaining that I will ask her to repeat it for me later "because I want to see how good your memory is"). The questioning should develop naturally from the opening remarks, and so far as possible take the form of a normal conversation.

The interview will deal with personal details such as the patient's age, date of birth, address, etc., and general matters. Wilson and Brass[2] have shown that a very short series of questions can detect, and roughly measure, intellectual impairment in old people living at home. Their 10 questions were, in brief: Town? Address? Date? Month? Year? Age? Year of birth? Month of birth? Prime Minister? Previous Prime Minister? The important thing is to ask the questions, and never simply to assume the answers, and to record the results, for comparison with future (or previous) testing. Finally, simple tests of cortical function—dysphasia and dyspraxia—should be made.

Basis of Management

At the end of the assessment, as well as having a good idea of the mental state, the doctor should be able to answer the following questions, on which the subsequent management largely rests:

Does the patient live alone?

How long since she was "normal" and competent? Was the change in her sudden, or gradual?

What has been the course of disability since then—steady or intermittent?

Is the patient mobile? Does she go out of the house?

What can she do for herself—toilet, wash, dress, clean, shop, cook?

What odd or undesirable behaviour—Does she wander? Is she incontinent?

Is she up at night? Does she make paranoid accusations? Is she aggressive or destructive?

What resources—relatives, friends, money—are available?

What services are already concerned?

WHICH CONSULTANT TO CALL?

If further specialist help is needed either in the home assessment or for possible hospital admission, the psychiatrist should be called when the problem is primarily one of behaviour disturbance. When it is primarily one of physical illness or decrepitude the geriatrician should be called. This division of responsibilities has recently been codified in the Government Memorandum on *Services for Mental Illness Related to Old Age*. One test of the quality of a district service for old people is that it should not matter too much if the "wrong" specialist is called, because geriatrician and psychiatrist will be used to working together and to taking patients from each other.

When even with the aid of a specialist the home assessment does not enable one to decide whether the disability is primarily medical or psychiatric, or when it appears that further assessment or care will need both general medical and psychiatric skills, the patient may be admitted to a "psychogeriatric assessment unit", or "joint patient unit". Unfortunately, few such units exist at present, but probably there will be more.

INVESTIGATIONS

In most cases a diagnosis of dementia, senile or arteriosclerotic, can be made at home. The history in an elderly person of progressive deterioration over months or years is so typical that when it coincides with the clinical findings, both physical and mental, the diagnosis can be regarded as conclusive. Nor is it necessary in such patients to pursue elaborate investigations designed to find out one of the rare and so-called reversible causes of dementia, when clinical evidence of them (for example, anaemia, hypothyroidism, papilloedema, or other abnormal neurological signs) are not in evidence. The most fashionable "reversible" causes of dementia are hypothyroidism, vitamin B_{12} deficiency, and normal pressure hydrocephalus, but when theie is established dementia with a long history of progressive deterioration treatment of the first two is most unlikely to benefit the mental state of the patient at all; of the third, with its triad of dementia, gait disturbance, and incontinence—which should be considered especially when there is a history of subarachnoid haemorrhage or meningitis—the same pessimistic view may ultimately prove to be justified, and there is the added hazard of the remedial operation. In most patients, who will be mostly in their 80s, home assessment will be sufficient to reach a conclusion, and the issue will then turn on management rather than on further investigation.

Further Observations or Fuller Investigations

In the following groups the history and intial examination should not alone be regarded as conclusive diagnosis of dementia.

(1) Patients in whom there is a history of depressive illness, or any features suggestive of depression.

(2) All patients under the age of 70, except when there is an obvious cerebrovascular cause.

(3) Patients of any age, whose history is atypical or uncertain—for example, too short a course, an apparently rapid fulminating course, an atypically intermittent course.

(4) Patients in whom there are other unusual features—for example, recent significant injury, intercurrent illness, alcoholism, drug abuse—and patients with unexplained physical findings, or whose physical state is strikingly incongruous with their mental state, or whose mental state on examination is greatly at variance with what would be expected from the history.

(5) Patients in whom "one has the feel" that they are somehow "not right". This is hardly a helpful category to others, but psychiatrists working in the field of psychogeriatrics will know what I mean. These patients may turn out to be depressed. Some may attribute this category to imprecision of thinking or observation, and they may be right.

Further investigation is likely to comprise blood count and sedimentation rate; Wasserman or equivalent test; blood sugar and urea levels and electrolytes; urine analysis; chest and skull x-ray films; protein-bound iodine (or other more specific tests of thyroid function); serum vitamin B_{12} and folate; liver tests will be appropriate if there is any evidence of alcoholism. The test for syphilis in the elderly is nowadays done more for tradition's sake than for the likelihood that it will yield a result of significance for the patient: the occasional positive WR picked up in this way is almost always incidental to rather than the cause of the dementia and is one of the "persistent positives" which occur among thoroughly treated cases of syphilis. Most of the above are tests which we perform routinely on inpatients, but of course most of our inpatients are not demented, and many have acute confusional states; other laboratory tests may be made necessary by specific findings.

Psychological tests may sometimes help when there are specific deficits, though in our experience they are more helpful in providing a base-line against which to measure change. Electroencephalography is likely merely to confirm the presence of diffuse abnormality in severely demented patients, and to be normal in the mild or uncertain case, though this and radioactive brain scan or ultrasonic techniques may be useful if there is a suspicion of a cerebral tumour. Examination of the cerebrospinal fluid is only rarely necessary in demented elderly patients; grounds for suspecting a brain tumour or syphilis are the main indications (and a sample of cerebrospinal fluid will anyway be available if pneumonencephalography is performed).

When to do Air Studies

In the absence of evidence suggesting space-occupying pathology (when angiography would sometimes be the appropriate technique) the value of pneumoencephalography is almost wholly limited to confirming the presence of brain atrophy. Such confirmation may reassure doctors and relatives and so give confidence in planning further management, and on these grounds may be justified, at least in the "younger" geriatric patient. But one should remember in these circumstances that one is ordering the investigation more for confirmation than in the hope of revealing remediable pathology.

The procedure is unpleasant and not without risk. In the investigation of dementia in the elderly air studies should be restricted to:

(1) Patients under 70, or perhaps 75, in whom there is no obvious cerebrovascular cause for their dementia to confirm the presence of cortical atrophy;

(2) Patients in whom despite negative findings in other tests, there is still some reason to suggest a space-occupying mass; and

(3) Patients in whom there is cause to suspect the presence of "communicating hydrocephalus".

These comments refer to patients with a typical history and clinical picture of dementia, and not to acutely confused patients who may require exhaustive investigation, which will indeed often reveal remediable lesions. All those patients in whom we have found tumours, subdural haematomas, cysts, etc., have had clinical features which have led us to investigate more fully. I do myself not recall any patient who, having been routinely investigated with pneumoencephalography merely on the grounds of being under 70, has surprised us by revealing some unsuspected remediable condition; and it is fair to assume that the results of performing these procedures on older typically demented patients would be no different.

REFERENCES

[1] Walton, H. J., Drewery, J., and Phillip, A. E., *British Medical Journal*, 1964, 2, 744.
[2] Wilson, L. A., and Brass, W., *Age and Ageing*, 1973, 2, 92.

Dementia in the Elderly: Management

BY

TOM ARIE

MOST demented people are at home. Dementia greatly increases the likelihood that an old person will eventually need institutional care, but it is not in itself grounds for removal from home; except where short-term hospital admission for investigation or treatment is necessary, the issue turns on the resources and tolerance available outside the hospital as much as on the disease itself. Thus in most cases the doctor's job is to see that all available medical and social sources of help are deployed, and to co-ordinate and monitor their provision.

CAN THE PATIENT BE MANAGED AT HOME?

The old person who lives alone poses the biggest problem. The available services are rarely able to offer anything approaching continuing around-the-clock care, yet such old people often have to be admitted not because they need heavy care, but simply because they need someone to "be around" to keep an eye on them most of the time—to reassure or gently to restrain if they start to wander out of the house. If they cannot have this care at home, then it is residential, not hospital care that they need. But old people who are being looked after by relatives or friends may pose equally taxing problems. Sometimes the burden of disability or behaviour disorder is such that the doctor may feel it his duty to try to persuade a devoted family to accept that their parent is beyond their reasonable capacity to cope, and to help them with their guilt at accepting institutional care. The cost of caring for an aged relative in terms of stress, and even of lasting damage to such families may be clearer to the doctor than to the family, who may find it hard to confess it to themselves or to each other.

More often the old person can well continue to be looked after at home; and relatives and friends will often want to continue to do so. Often it is not the immediate burden that makes families despair, but the prospect of carrying on indefinitely without relief, or without even the expectation of a holiday—or for that matter, without some recognition by others of the size of the burden which they are carrying. Often the whole burden of caring for an aged parent seems to be carried by only one among many brothers and sisters, commonly for reasons which are obscure or derive from long-standing family feuds. In these cases the child who is doing the caring may voice so much resentment towards the brothers and sisters who "don't want to know", that the

104

doctor thinks that the resentment is harder for them to bear than the burden itself. The family's attitude to an old person seems often to derive more from her past personality and behaviour towards them, than from the objective burden of her dementia: in a word, whether they like her.

Many families who do not want to give up the care of the old person need reassurance that their difficulties are appreciated, and not taken for granted, and "therapeutic listening" will go a long way. But often families are unaware that welfare services exist at all, or, for example, that the old person can have guaranteed periods of relief-admission to hospital or old people's home and that their holiday arrangements can be underwritten by booking a temporary admission. Often too the behaviour problems can be greatly mitigated by medical measures, which will be discussed later.

If the decision is for hospital admission the family must be clear why the patient is being admitted—whether it is for care and not for "treatment", or whether it is for short-term investigation only. Sometimes the family's hopes prove stronger even than careful attempts to explain. In a good unit, however demented the patient, she is likely when first admitted to go to an assessment ward, and only very rarely will a commitment to permanent hospital care be made at the time of admission.

Is Day Care Likely to Help?

Day care may help families and may give an opportunity further to assess or treat the patient. But demented old people generally take poorly to being moved from place to place and easily become confused and this may limit the feasibility of day care for some patients, just as it often restricts the appropriateness of "rotating" admission, which is such a source of help to many families looking after physically sick old people.

There are often transport difficulties; it may be impossible to pick up a patient, even if she can be got up and ready, before the family leave for work; and at the other end of the day relatives still have the old person arriving home at about the same time as they themselves get back weary from work. It may be possible to let the family have some respite in the evenings by offering to keep the day-patient until after they had have had their supper, and giving her hers in hospital. This generally depends on the family being able to make their own arrangement for collecting her, since transport is rarely available at this time. Many of these problems are solved when the day hospital has its own minibus and driver. Another scheme which at least one enterprising local authority is trying out is a "granny-sitting" service in the evenings at residential homes; by arrangement with the matron, families wishing to go out in the evening may leave an aged relative watching the television with other old people—but, again, confused old people may become still more confused by such temporary changes of surroundings.

CAN THE PATIENT MANAGE HER FINANCIAL AFFAIRS?

An important practical aspect of the care of demented old people, often forgotten, is the legal one. A demented person is most unlikely to be able to appreciate the nature of her affairs, still less to look after them, and if there are any substantial assets the family should be advised to contact the Court of Protection. In these circumstances a Power of Attorney is inappropriate because the old person is unlikely to be capable of understanding its significance. The approach to the Court of Protection may be made through a solicitor, or to the Personal Applications Branch*. Occasionally it may be the doctor's duty to contact the Court, if he has reason to believe that a demented person is being financially exploited.

INFORMAL OR COMPULSORY ADMISSION?

About 15% of our own admitted patients with organic psychosyndromes come into hospital under compulsion, almost all of them under Section 25 of the Mental Health Act. It is impossible to give hard-and-fast advice on when the use of these powers is justified and the decision can be a taxing one; paradoxically perhaps, I have, very rarely, used an Order to bring in for a temporary relief admission a demented old person being cared for by her family, yet refused to do so in respect of a demented old person who lives alone and constitutes some danger to herself.

This is the result of using the following general criterion: If the old person's unwillingness to enter hospital is, in the light of at least a reasonable awareness of the consequences for herself and for others, due to a clear wish to remain at home, it is rarely justifiable to remove her compulsorily. But if her refusal is the result of lack of insight or delusional attitudes to her predicament—that is, if her refusal is itself the result of her mental disorder—removal is probably justified if she cannot reasonably be cared for at home. By this criterion an old lady living on her own who has perhaps had several falls or even wandered out into the road on occasion, but who has a reasonable grasp of her situation and often indicates her wishes forcibly by some such phrase as "I want to die in my own home" should be left at home, though attempts to persuade her that she needs more care should continue.

If a psychiatrist, balancing the risks in relation to the patient's welfare and civil rights, decides against compulsory admission, it is reasonable

* Staffordshire House, Store Street, London, W.C.1. telephone 01-636 6877.

for the general practitioner to expect him to make his reasons clear in writing and to share the responsibility, for such a lady may well come to harm at home, or she may wander out in front of a passing car (and the predicament of the potential passing motorist who may have her death on his conscience must be considered too).

By contrast a perhaps less demented old person who is nevertheless wholly dependent on others for her personal functioning, who rarely moves from her room, yet who insists that she is entirely independent, that she does her own shopping, etc., may justify compulsory admission. But such cases are difficult and always sad.

In deciding on compulsory admission because of the hazards at home, one has to weigh also the hazards of an enforced change of surroundings, which is often followed by greater confusion and mysterious decline and death. Clear thinking on these matters demands that the interests of the patient and the interests of other people be distinguished, though each has a right to be considered; errors of both logic and humanity can occur when the one is confused with the other.

No patient (old or young) should ever be denied admission to a medical (or surgical) bed when that is what they need, merely because they come under compulsion; this was the clear intention of the Mental Health Act of 1959. Special nursing provision may have to be made for such patients in a general ward, but more commonly they pose few problems. The belief that a confused old person admitted under compulsory powers is likely to be more disturbed than one who has come informally is understandable but false, and it is rarely these patients that upset medical wards.

WHAT SUPPORTIVE SERVICES ARE NEEDED?

An account of the supportive services would make an article in itself, and the unevenness of their availability in different areas is notorious. I list only the main ones; fuller advice should always be available from the area office of the social services department.

(1) Support and surveillance may be sought from social workers, health visitors, district nurses, and occasionally specially appointed "geriatric visitors".

(2) Home helps and home meals are obtained through the social services department or on direct application to the organizers of the particular service.

(3) Modifications to the home, appliances such as walking aids or commodes, and disposable incontinence pads or sheets (and in some areas a laundry service) may be arranged through the social worker or in some cases direct with the health department, or with the aid of the health visitor.

(4) Chiropody services are in relatively short supply, as are home

physiotherapy and home occupational therapy; in some areas these are unobtainable.

(5) Local authorities may run day centres, often with transport, but these are not always suitable for, or willing to receive, confused old people; only in a minority of areas are there special day centres for the elderly confused. Many local authorities will accept old people for the day care at old people's homes.

(6) In most areas there is an Old People's Welfare Association, which organizes activities such as visiting, clubs, competitions, etc., using lay volunteers.

(7) The local authority may sometimes be able to organize holidays even for quite demented old people.

(8) Some demented old people may be so dependent as to qualify for either the full, or the partial Attendance Allowance.

RESIDENTIAL ACCOMMODATION

Residential accommodation is the responsibility of the social services department under Part III of the National Assistance Act and the extent and type of provision are extremely variable up and down the country. Some local authorities have special homes for the "elderly mentally confused", and, though these have recently been criticized, I believe that well-designed and well-run ones are the most appropriate way of meeting the needs of some demented old people. But most demented old people living in residential care are in ordinary old people's homes, and dementia itself (as opposed to severe behaviour disorder or severe nursing dependency) should not disqualify an old person for a place in such a home. Doctors who are in the habit of visiting old people's homes will not need telling that anything from a third to over a half of residents there are appreciably demented. The Government has urged local authorities to expand residential provision, but it is certain to remain in short supply almost everywhere. Lists of private residential homes should be available from social services departments; some are excellent, others frightful.

Warden-supervised "sheltered" accommodation comes under the housing department, and control of sheltered housing and residential accommodation are thus unfortunately separated administratively. In fact, sheltered accommodation is almost never appropriate for a demented old person, unless he or she is to live with a well-preserved spouse.

MEDICATION

Depression, intercurrent illnesses, and contributory ailments and disabilities must of course all be treated in their own right. There are no specific drugs for dementia; drugs for which it is claimed that they improve cerebral blood supply or oxygen utilization have not yet been proved to be of practical value and I do not use them, though this may change in the light of new drugs or convincing evaluations.

Tranquillizers

The staple drugs in the management of behaviour disturbance in demented old people are the tranquillizers and there is little evidence that any one is much better than any other.

It is best to become accustomed to one or two drugs, and I prefer promazine because it is not as potent weight for weight as the other phenothazines, and its dosage can thus be more exactly adjusted; when heavier dosage is required I use thioridazine or chlorpromazine. though with the latter jaundice is not a negligible risk. Some units make more extensive use than we do of the butyrophenone haloperidol. The tranquillizing value of chlormethiazole has not yet been established.

Often old people prefer "medicine" to tablets, and syrup is thus sometime acceptable when tablets are not; and liquid is harder to hide in the mouth and subsequently spit out than are tablets, and cannot be hoarded in pockets or under pillows.

The important thing about tranquillizing regimens is that they should be planned and titrated against the patient's needs. So used they can be an important part of the management, not only of confusion but of paranoid phenomena and of the repetitive questioning and overactivity which can drive relatives to distraction. There is no place for shutting the stable door after the horse has bolted—for large doses to be given only when the grossly disturbed behaviour has already occurred. In such circumstances one is likely merely to make the patient unconscious, or even to make her more confused. One must try to forestall the disturbance, without making the patient dopey. This means taking a careful history of the pattern and circumstances in which the disturbed behaviour most often occurs.

The commonest problem is nocturnal restlessness, and an increased dose of the tranquillizing drug at bedtime together with a hypnotic such as nitrazepam will often give a night's sleep to both the patient and her relatives. It is traditional not to use barbiturates as hypnotics for confused old people, since they are said readily to produce either increased confusion or excitement.

Depot Fluphenazines

There is a very limited place for the depot preparations of fluphenazine either in the decanoate or enanthate form.

The trouble with these drugs, which need to be given only once every three or four weeks (and which in old people should generally be given in about half the dose of younger people and if necessary more frequently), is that they have a high incidence of dystonic and depressant side effects. Once the injection is given the effect cannot be wholly reversed until the drugs has been metabolized. Old people with extrapyramidal disease, or very decrepit old people, are thus unlikely to tolerate these drugs, but we find that a few relatively robust demented patients may be much helped by them. When phenothiazine medication is associated with Parkinsonian side effects, an anti-Parkinsonian drug such as orphenadrine, 50 mg thrice daily, is given concurrently—though anti-Parkinsonian drugs, notably benzhexol, are themselves prone to cause confusion in old people. When it cannot be controlled by general measures or oral drugs acute confusion or excitement almost always responds to intramuscular injection of 50 or 100 mg of chlorpromazine.

Too heavy transquillizing (or antidepressant) medication may make a confused patient more confused: drug regimens must be reviewed often, and reduction of medication may be more effective than additions.

Vitamins have no proved value in dementia unless there is evidence of a deficiency state; but it makes sense to give them to old people who have been living alone and not eating well.

OTHER PRACTICAL MEASURES

There are no easy answers to problems such as wandering or incontinence. Often drug control of night-time restlessness can fortify the family by ensuring a night's sleep for everyone. But simple practical measures may go a long way: thus, fitting a lock on a door may stop aimless wandering on to the street, and so enable the family temporarily to leave an otherwise contented old person alone; a change from more dangerous gas or oil to safer electric appliances can diminish obvious dangers; an approach by the doctor or social worker to a friend or local teenager, whom the family may be shy to ask, may give regular periods of help to enable relatives to do shopping, or to have an evening out. Incontinence of urine is dealt with in a later article, but of faecal incontinence it should be remembered that it is most often due to a remediable cause, such as diarrhoea or impaction, and periodic enemas may solve the problem.

CONCLUSION

Old people with failing brains have three main needs: for security, because their capacity to function far outstrips their capacity to adapt to change; for stimulation, because dementia, especially when restricted mobility and sensory privation in the form of deafness or blindness are added to it, makes the world a frightening and lonely place, in which withdrawal and apathy may be the way of least resistance; and for patience, because old people are slow, but time and again will astonish one by their capacity to "get there in the end"—indeed, they are often "there" from the start, and it is their attendants who are too hurried to get there with them.

These needs are not of course confined to the demented elderly, but are among the basic needs of all of us, but the disabilities of the demented may make their needs more urgent, and their lack of inhibition may make more direct the efforts to satisfy them. The "attention-seeking" behaviour of old people, their wandering, and their incontinence, may in part at least become intelligible, and so perhaps more manageable, if seen against the background of these needs.

But no amount of understanding can make the care of demented old people easy, and the doctor and social worker must beware of attempting to "interpret away" the heavy realities of caring for these severely disabled old people. I hope that this review will be of some practical help, but I should not disagree with the view that not all human problems have their solutions.

FURTHER READING

Sources for statements other than personal opinions will be found in the following, which also provide a way into the now growing literature of dementia.

The British Journal of Hospital Medicine of March 1969 contains five review articles on various aspects of dementia.

Recent Developments in Psychogeriatrics, ed. by D. W. K. Kay and A. Walk. London, Royal Medico-Psychological Association, 1971, is a valuable symposium.

Sir Martin Roth's review of "The Psychogeriatric Problem" in *Approaches to Action*, ed. by G. McLachlan. London, Oxford University Press for Nuffield Provincial Hospitals Trust, 1972. Another chapter in the same volume gives an account of our own psychiatric service for old people at Goodmayes Hospital.

Felix Post's *The Clinical Psychiatry of Late Life*. Oxford, Pergamon, 1965, and the chapter on *Mental Disorders in the Aged* (effectively a short text book in itself) in Mayer-Gross, Slater, and Roth's *Clinical Psychiatry*, 3rd edn. London, Bailliere, Tindall and Cassell, 1969, are authoritative accounts of geriatric psychiatry.

Diseases of the Motor System

BY

W. J. NICHOLSON

THE Registrar General's *Statistical Review of England and Wales for the Year 1970* shows that 19% of all deaths in the over-65s were directly attributed to diseases of the nervous system. In addition, the 4% of all deaths in the same age group attributed to diseases of the arteries must include a proportion with central nervous system involvement. Mortality figures reflect morbidity (see fig.); every geriatric department contains more patients in this disease category than in any other. Though patients over 65 constitute only 12% of the total population, they occupy over one-third of the total NHS beds—or a total of roughly 80,000 excluding psychiatric hospitals. Taken together, these facts indicate that elderly patients with diseases of the central nervous system must make formidable demands on the resources of the NHS. Moreover, with an annual rise of 100,000 in the over-65s this demand must continue to increase.

DISEASE OF THE PYRAMIDAL SYSTEM

By far the commonest disease of the central nervous system encountered is a stroke, varying from a disabling hemiplegia to a transient ischaemic cerebral episode with rapid recovery. A stroke with paralysis warranting admission to hospital is more common than acute appendicitis; a general practitioner with a list of 3,000 will see five new strokes each year and will have a similar number of disabled stroke survivors on his list. The annual stroke incidence is about two per 1,000 of the total population—which means 110,000 new stroke presentations each year in England and Wales. Three-quarters of all stroke patients are over the age of 65. In the United Kingdom 130,000 patients have appreciable impairment from a stroke and 93,000 of these are severely handicapped.[1]

The onset of a stroke due to cerebral thrombosis or embolism is usually first noticed after a period of sleep or rest. The patient may rise from bed to go to the lavatory and promptly falls owing to paresis of the leg. Relatives may become alarmed because the patient is vacant and confused after an afternoon nap; when the doctor arrives the patient appears normal again. This latter episode is typical of transient ischaemic cerebral episodes, which may recur with frequency.

The patient with a major stroke has motor weakness of both the arm and leg; initially there is flaccid muscle tone with sluggish reflexes, but

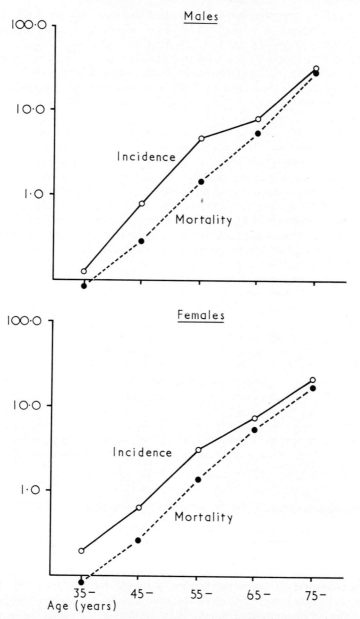

Semilogarithmic plot by age and sex of estimates of incidence and mortality in the Oxford Record Linkage area in 1963 for all types of stroke combined. (Acheson, R. M., and Fairbairn, A. S., *British Medical Journal*, 1970, **2**, 621.)

after a few days the tone increases and the jerks become brisk. The plantar response is extensor. The motor weakness is rarely equal in both arm and leg, one limb having more pareses than the other, depending on the arterial territory maximally involved. Occlusion of the anterior cerebral artery results in maximum motor weakness in the contralateral leg; occlusion of the middle cerebral artery produces paralysis maximum in contralateral arm and face, with aphasia should the dominant hemisphere be involved.

The last two decades have seen a revolution in the management and rehabilitation of the patient with a stroke.[2] In the early weeks after a stroke the mortality is about 50%; of the survivors, half regain independence in daily living activities outside hospital. Beyond question the best results are obtained by admitting all patients to special stroke units, where ancillary forces can be concentrated and where the patient's morale is maintained by a team spirit with patients pacing each other in the race to recovery; this is the best therapy to combat fatalism.

Most patients with uncomplicated hemiplegia spend two to three months retraining to stand and walk. Improvement in motor power can still be expected for up to eight months. Patients who progress to the point of social rehabilitation at home must be followed up for at least two years in the outpatient department or in day hospital. Careful neurological analysis of every stroke patient pays great dividends in successful rehabilitation. For most patients recovery is slow but persistent; for those with delayed recovery it is imperative to identify the barriers to progress;[3] these include dysphasia, cortical sensory deficit, impaired muscle joint position, or an associated psychiatric disturbance. A discussion with the physiotherapist and occupational therapist on the reasons for delayed recovery is essential.

When discharge is planned it is prudent for the occupational therapist to visit the house and advise on what help for the handicapped[4] is required in the way of a supporting rail, ramp, or aids to daily living in the kitchen.

Pseudobulbar Palsy

During recovery from a stroke a second cerebrovascular accident may occur on the opposite side. If both areas of vascular occlusion are in the region of the internal capsule then pseudobulbar palsy may result. Pseudobulbar palsy occurs in patients who are hypertensive and in characterized by emotional lability, a spastic tongue, brisk jaw jerk, and an upper motor neurone lesion in all four limbs; death results from aspiration pneumonia. The emotional lability is distressing for patient and relatives but alleviation can be obtained with imipramine[5] or amitriptylline.[6]

Brain Stem Ischaemia

Vascular insufficiency or occlusion in the posterior cerebral circulation results in one of the brain stem syndromes. Here the patient is prostrated with severe giddiness, double vision, vomiting, and ataxia. On examination, there is nystagmus, intention tremor in the ipsilateral limbs, and numbness in the ipsilateral face and contralateral side of the body. Ipsilateral involvement of a cranial nerve may be present. Despite the alarming onset the prognosis is good.

Motor Neurone Disease

As in younger people, motor neurone disease is characterized by weakness and wasting in all four limbs, fasciculation being maximum in the shoulder and pelvic girdles; all limb reflexes are brisk, the plantars are extensor and there is no sphincter disturbance. However, unlike the younger age groups, the prognosis is much more favourable with survival for more than a decade. Even with bulbar involvement there is a relatively better prognosis.[7]

DISEASE OF THE EXTRAPYRAMIDAL SYSTEM

In 1817 an East London general practitioner, Dr. James Parkinson, published *An Essay on the Shaking Palsy*, giving a lucid description of the clinical manifestation of disease of the extrapyramidal system. Every general practice contains several patients with Parkinsonism easily remembered both by their appearance and by the "repeat prescription" list. Parkinsonism or paralysis agitans is due to disease of the basal ganglia. Primary degeneration of unknown aetiology is the commonest cause, with degeneration secondary to vascular disease or to encephalitis lethargica being much less frequent. Drugs can cause Parkinsonism, the chief offenders being methyl dopa, reserpine, chlorpromazine, and the phenothiazines; haloperidol is notable for causing the rapid production of Parkinsonian features. Parkinsonism caused by drugs is dose-dependent. Carbon monoxide intoxication and manganese poisoning are often quoted but rarely seen aetiologies of Parkinsonism, but most geriatric department have an ex-boxer with this disease.

Clinically Parkinsonism is recognised at a glance, from the fixed expressionless gaze, infrequent blinking, and festinating walk in small steps with bent attitude. Roughly half the patients exhibit the coarse compound tremor, which may affect any or all of the limbs as well as the jaw. The tremor is present at rest but disappears when the patient voluntarily uses the limb or falls asleep; anxiety worsens the tremor. The limb reflexes are normal. The postencephalitic type of Parkinsonism, with seborrhoeic skin, drooling saliva, and oculogyric crisis, is rarely seen because there are now few survivors of the 1920 epidemic.

Treatment

The introduction of L-dopa represented a major advance in therapeutics. Unfortunately, not all patients are suitable for this therapy; it is a good working rule that to benefit a patient must be clear in the head and be prepared to tolerate the nausea during the "build up" until the improvement is obvious.[8] Initial dosage must be small— for example, L-dopa 0·25 mg thrice daily after food. Dosage may be increased by 0·5 g every fourth day, but if nausea and vomiting cannot be tolerated then reversion to a smaller dose with a slower "build up" must be made. Nausea may also be reduced by using one of the slow release preparation such as Broca Dopa temp tabs. Months rather than weeks should be the aim in reaching the optimum dosage of 5 g daily, always remembering that maximum improvement may take six months to occur. Once a patient has increased mobility, a sense of well-being and renewed vigour for daily living activities she will not hesitate to persist with L-dopa. Patients frequently receive tonics in the form of polyvitamin preparations; pyridoxine (vitamin B_6) cancels the clinical action of L-dopa and since it is present in many vitamin mixtures care must be taken to avoid it. Like all powerful drugs, L-dopa has serious side effects: depression, anxiety, or confusion may force withdrawal of the drug. Abnormal involuntary movements may occur affecting the face, neck, and spinal muscles or even causing rhythmic movements of the abdominal wall. Cardiac arrhythmia and hypotension are hazards in patients with pre-existing coronary artery disease. Fortunately all the toxic effects are dose-dependent. The introduction of L-dopa decarboxylase inhibitors promises the maximum benefit of L-dopa with minimum toxic effects.

Because of the danger of hypertensive crisis monoamine oxidase inhibitor drugs must never be administered at the same time as L-dopa. Sympathomimetic agents must also be avoided.

Conventional anticholinergic drugs such as orphenadrine 50 mg thrice daily may safely be given to supplement therapy with L-dopa. In patients unsuitable for L-dopa therapy the anticholinergic drugs may still be useful, but it is important to remember that they can precipitate acute glaucoma or acute urinary retention. Amantadine has beeen disappointing in treatment of the patient with Parkinsonism but is always worth a trial where the other two lines of therapy have failed.

Hemiballismus

A vascular lesion of the subthalamic nucleus results in sudden onset of violent choreic movements in the contralateral half of the body. The violence of the movements rapidly exhausts the patient and involvement of the pharyngeal muscles may result in aspiration pneumonia. Tetrabenazine is effective in relieving the movements but the movements can be abolished only with thalamotomy.

LOWER MOTOR NEURONE LESIONS

Polyneuropathy represents the commonest lower motor neurone lesion of old age and is characterized by bilateral flaccid muscle weakness maximum in the distal limb muscles, always worse in the legs. There may also be sensory loss of the stocking-and-glove types. Most cases of peripheral neuropathy are mixed motor and sensory. Asymmetry is most unusual in either motor or sensory component.

The clinical signs are weakness, sluggish or absent reflexes, wasting of the muscles, and tenderness of the muscles and soles of the feet; tenderness is a prominent feature of alcoholic neuropathy but may occur in the acute stage of any neuropathy. The sensory loss usually involves all modalities of sensation. Plantar responses are flexor or absent.

Diabetes mellitus represents the most likely cause of a polyneuropathy in any old person. Routine urine testing cannot rule out the diagnosis —nor can one estimation of the blood sugar level. A glucose tolerance test should be performed in all cases when both urine tests and blood sugar levels are inconclusive. Most elderly diabetics are obese and management of the polyneuropathy aims at arresting its progress by good diabetic control, preferably by diet supplemented if required by a sulphonylurea or a diguanide preparation. Diabetic peripheral neuropathy may be purely sensory and may affect only muscle joint and vibration sensations—hence the description of this condition as "diabetic pseudotabes". These patients may develop perforating ulcers in the feet and, with vascular impairment, great care must be taken in chiropody.

Polyneuropathy may be the presenting manifestation of a carcinoma, especially carcinoma of the bronchus, occurring long before the primary neoplasm is obvious. Herpes zoster, even a mild and limited infection, may be complicated by polyneuropathy.

Deficiency of vitamin B_{12} either in Addisonian pernicious anaemia or in a malabsorption syndrome may result in polyneuropathy, but this may be associated with posterior column signs to cause subacute combined degeneration. Systemic therapy with vitamin B_{12} will reverse the lesion in the lower motor neurone but will only arrest the lesion in the posterior column.

The extent of alcoholism is probably underestimated in elderly women, who prefer to avoid drinking in pubs. In addition to peripheral neuropathy, these patients may develop a gross memory defect or become very confused: hence Korsakoff's psychosis may be diagnosed as senile dementia. The value of Parenterovite is questionable, but it seems to provide psychotherapy for the officiating physician and a jolt to the sobering patient.

Drugs which may cause polyneuropathy are the inorganic arsenicals, gold, sulphonamides, nitrofurantoin, and isoniazid.

Patients with polyneuropathy of any aetiology will become disabled and unable to walk. While the primary aetiology is being treated ambulation must be maintained or regained with physiotherapy.

REFERENCES

[1] Harris, A. I., Cox, E., and Smith, C. R. W., *Handicapped and Impaired in Great Britain*, part 1. London, H.M.S.O., 1971.
[2] Adams, G. F., *Gerontologia Clinica*, 1967, **9**, 285.
[3] Adams, G. F., and Hurwitz, L. J., *Lancet*, 1963, **2**, 533.
[4] Hurwitz, L. J., *British Medical Journal*, 1969, **3**, 699.
[5] Lawson, I. R. and MacLeod, R. D. M., *British Journal of Psychiatry*, 1969 **115**, 281.
[6] Hamilton, L. D., *Clinical Medicine*, 1966, **73**, No. 9, 49.
[7] Hodkinson, H. M., *Age and Ageing*, **1**, 182.
[8] Godwin-Austin, R. B., Tomlinson, E. B., Frears, C. C., and Kok, H. W. L., *Lancet*, 1969, **2**, 165.

Accidental Hypothermia

BY

A. N. EXTON-SMITH

IT is generally considered that a hypothermic state exists when the *deep* body temperature falls below an arbitrarily defined limit of 35°C (or 95°F). The term accidental hypothermia is used to imply that the lowering of the body temperature is unintentional and it has to be distinguished from hypothermia induced for the purposes of medical or surgical treatment.

INCIDENCE

The British Medical Association Committee on Accidental Hypothermia in the Elderly,[1] after reviewing the descriptions of cases published in Britain up to the early 1960s, concluded that there was no accurate information on the incidence of the condition. The hospital reports indicated that very few cases were recognized before admission and elderly people with hypothermia suffered a high mortality. Death resulted from the often serious nature of the underlying disease as well as from the effects of hypothermia itself.

The Registrar General's returns of death certificates indicate that only about 100 fatal cases are reported annually.[2] These figures are at variance with those reported in the survey conducted by the Royal College of Physicians.[3] Ten hospital groups co-operated in the investigation and during the three months 1 February to 30 April 1965 it was found that 126 patients had rectal temperatures of 35°C or less on admission, representing 0·68% of all admissions. It was estimated that there could have been 9,000 patients admitted to hospitals in England and Wales with hypothermia during the three winter months, and 42% of these patients were over the age of 65. The true incidence is probably much higher than this, especially among the elderly, since the survey did not include those patients treated at home in many of whom hypothermia passes unrecognized.

RELATION BETWEEN BODY TEMPERATURE AND ENVIRONMENTAL CONDITIONS

The results of the first large-scale national survey of body temperatures of old people in Great Britain living at home were reported by Fox and his colleagues in 1973.[2] The investigation was based on measurements made on 1,020 people of 65 years and over during the

119

first three months of 1972. In 754 cases (75%) the room temperatures the old people were at or below 18·3°C (65°F)—the minimum recommended by the Parker Morris report on council housing—and in 10% the morning living-room temperatures were very cold, at or below 12·0°C. The deep body temperatures in the morning and evening were measured by the Uritemp technique.[4] In about 10% of subjects the deep body temperatures were below 35·5°C ("low" group) and these were considered to be at risk of developing hypothermia. In comparison with a "normal" group (36·0°C and above), not only were they less successful in conserving body heat—as shown by their inability to maintain an adequate core/shell temperature gradient—but they also had a proportionately lower body heat content. The high prevalence of low room temperatures and of low body temperatures in the morning clearly indicated the need for measures to protect the individual from cold exposure at night. Disturbingly many individuals whose temperatures were in the "low" group were already receiving supplementary benefits, and yet only 3% of these pensioners were receiving an extra fuel allowance.

AETIOLOGY

The main causes of accidental hypothermia may be grouped under two headings:

Exogenous Factors

Exposure to cold is an over-riding cause, and there is a clear relation between the incidence of accidental hypothermia and a low environmental temperature. A common story is of an old person who falls after attempting to get out of bed at night; he remains on the floor for several hours, often partly clad, and is discovered only the next day by a neighbour or a home help. Thus probably the exposure is longer when the old person lives alone and is socially isolated. Very many cases, however, occur with lesser degrees of exposure, while the old person is in bed at night apparently well covered. In these instances insufficient body heat is being generated, so that even good external insulation is ineffective.

Endogenous Factors

Some degree of thermoregulatory failure is common in old age and the mechanisms for conserving body heat are impaired. Experiments on individual volunteers often show a poor shivering reaction in response to cold; while their deep body temperature is falling, older people are unaware of the cold exposure and do not complain of cold. Drugs acting on the nervous system can further impair physiological mechanisms. Thus chlorpromazine and other phenothiazines not only affect temperature regulation by abolishing shivering and causing vasodilatation, but they also lessen the patient's awareness of environmental hazards. The ingestion of alcohol, and a variety of sedatives, tranquillizers, and antidepressive drugs have all caused accidental hypothermia.

In addition to this impairment of temperature homoeostasis most severe examples of hypothermia in patients admitted to hospital have some underlying clinical condition. Almost any serious disorder may cause hypothermia but those commonly found are:

(1) Endocrine disorders: myxoedema and hypopituitarism in which the metabolic rate is lowered.

(2) Neurological disorders: especially cerebrovascular accident, which may not only be responsible for the initial fall causing exposure but, owing to the paralysis, for limiting the heat generated by muscular activity.

(3) Conditions associated with immobility—for example, stupor or coma from various causes, Parkinsonism, paraplegia, and chronic arthritis. These patients are often confined to bed and the lack of muscular activity leads to inadequate heat production.

(4) Mental impairment and confusional states: if such patients are not receiving sufficient supervision they may be unable to protect themselves from cold exposure.

(5) Severe infections and circulatory disturbances—for example, bronchopneumonia, cardiac infarction, and pulmonary embolism.

Thus a variety of acute and chronic conditions may be responsible, and in most cases of accidental hypothermia in the elderly both exogenous and endogenous factors operate in varying proportions.

CLINICAL FEATURES

A description of the clinical features is given in the reports of a series of cases treated in hospital by Duguid and her colleagues[5] and by Rosin and Exton-Smith.[6]

Appearance

The intense peripheral vasoconstriction leads to pallor of the skin, and when cyanosis is also present the patient has a pallid grey colour. There is puffiness of the face and this together with the slow cerebration and the husky voice may be thought to be due to myxoedema.

Nervous System

As the body temperature falls below 32°C clouding of consciousness, progressive confusion, and drowsiness develop. The patient's responses are slow and the reflexes are sluggish. Shivering is absent and below about 30°C it is replaced by a muscular hypertonus. This may lead to neck stiffness simulating meningism and to rigidity of the limbs. An involuntary flapping tremor in the arms and legs has been observed in some cases.[6]

Respiratory System

The respirations are slow and shallow. An appreciable fall in arterial oxygen saturation may occur as the result of this hypopnoea; the effect of anoxia on the tissue metabolism is one of the factors determining prognosis. Bronchopneumonia is nearly always present, but it may not be detected owing to the absence of the usual clinical signs.

Cardiovascular System

In response to cold the heart rate slows due to sinus bradycardia or to slow atrial fibrillation. In the early stages the blood pressure is maintained but a fall in blood pressure in spite of the intense periperal vasoconstriction is a bad prognostic sign. The electrocardiogram often shows some degree of heart block with lengthening of the PR interval and delay in intraventricular conduction. A pathognomonic sign is the appearance of a "J" wave with a characteristic deflection at the junction of the QRS and ST segments. These waves, which are usually best seen in V4, occur only in about a third of cases.

Alimentary System

Post-mortem examination often shows acute pancreatitis, but the clinical diagnosis is rarely made. The clouding of consciousness and the muscular rigidity of the abdominal wall due to hypothermia obscure the usual signs, but pancreatitis should be suspected if the patient is seen to wince when firm pressure is applied to the epigastrium. The serum amylase is raised in most severe cases of hypothermia.

MANAGEMENT

Patients with mild degrees of hypothermia (with a temperature just below 35°C) can sometimes be treated at home. The adverse social circumstances which led to the hypothermia often preclude home treatment, even in the less serious cases. When the deep body temperature is less than 32°C urgent admission is required since treatment can only be given in hospital.

There has for long been controversy about the best way of restoring normal body temperature. The dangers of rapid rewarming, which may cause circulatory collapse and an "after-drop" of the deep body temperature, are well known. It is therefore often advocated that there should be no active rewarming at all, the patient being lightly covered in a ward at an ambient temperature of 21°C and his temperature allowed to come up very slowly. The disadvantage of this method is that when there has already been long exposure to cold at home the period of hypothermia is greatly prolonged and irreversible changes in the tissues may take place. The incidence of complications and the late mortality are related to the duration of the hypothermia. There is need for further investigation of methods of rewarming, but the assessment of results using different methods of treatment is made difficult because prognosis is determined by the nature of the underlying disease as well as by the severity of hypothermia. It is now believed, however, that better results can be obtained by more rapid rewarming provided the patient is treated in an intensive care unit.

Most patients with severe hypothermia will require the following measures: (1) the administration of oxygen and the institution of intermittent positive pressure ventilation; (2) the insertion of a central venous catheter for the measurement of pressure and the administration of warm fluids; (3) the correction of dehydration and of metabolic acidosis; (4) the intravenous administration of hydrocortisone and a broad-spectrum antibiotic, which is given because bronchopneumonia often develops insidiously; and (5) the continuous or frequent monitoring of deep body temperature.

When accidential hypothermia is associated with barbiturate overdosage, perintoneal dialysis has been used successfully with the dual purpose of removing barbiturate from the blood stream and for rewarming the large vascular areas and organs of the abdomen. Only if there is a strong suspicion from the clinical history or laboratory evidence that the hypothermia is due to myxoedema should tri-iodothyronine be given. The dose used is small (10 μg eight to twelve hourly) since in high dosage myocardial infarction may be precipitated.

PREVENTIVE MEASURES

Recognition of Old People at Risk

Doctors and community nurses should pay particular attention to old people living in cold accommodation even though they say they do not feel the cold. The regular recording of deep body temperature either by means of a low-reading rectal thermometer or by the Uritemp technique, especially in those whose activities are restricted by chronic illness or disability, would be valuable. The Health Departments of some local authorities operate visiting schemes for those most at risk including the over 75s, those living alone (and very elderly couples living by themselves), the housebound, and the handicapped. Social workers can detect many unmet needs in isolated old people and they should be aware of the circumstances which lead to accidental hypo-thermia.

Heating

So far as possibly elderly people should be encouraged to install in their homes safe means of heating—for example, electric convector heaters and night storage heaters. The heating of the bedroom is just as important as that of the sitting room. In severe weather when it may be impossible to keep more than one room warm it is preferable to have adequate heat in the living room and to make up the bed in it. Since many old people in receipt of supplementary benefits are not receiving an extra fuel allowance (largely because they do not know about it), wider publicity needs to be given to the availability of extra heating allowances (see Department of Health and Social Security, *Provision for Heating, 1972.*[7])

Clothing and Blankets

Old people are sometimes found to be wearing unsuitable clothing, such as several felted woollen garments. For maximum comfort and warmth they should be advised that clothing needs to be light, closely woven, and not restricting. Similar comments also apply to bed clothes. Since many elderly people develop hypothermia at night, the protection against exposure to cold while they are in bed is important. Although there may be some resistance to the use of a new appliance an electric overblanket is very helpful. The conventional electric under-blanket should not be used because of hazards in incontinent patients. A low-voltage, low-wattage underblanket which is waterproof is being developed and this is proving to be an effective means of keeping old people warmer in bed.

Nutrition

Many of the factors which make a person at risk of developing hypothermia also lead to malnutrition, so the two conditions are some-times found together. The cost of extra fuel in winter may leave much less money to be spent on food. Many pensioners live on the borderline of malnutrition, and inadequate nutrition may occur just at the time when the energy needs of the body are greatest. It should be remembered however, that it is not necessarily the thin, seemingly undernourished old people who are predisposed to hypothermia since they are more likely to be active; it can occur in the obese inactive old person. In spite of the feeling of warmth which alcohol gives, old people should be warned that it increases heat loss from the body and is conducive to hypothermia. In winter there is a need for the general practitioner and health visitor to pay particular attention to the adequacy and nutrient content of the diet of old people.

CONCLUSION

For the diagnosis of accidental hypothermia the deep body temperature must be measured either by means of a rectal thermometer or by the Uritemp technique. The much wider use of low-reading thermometers by doctors and the community nursing services is essential, and there must be much greater awareness of the vulnerable groups in the elderly population. The early detection of accidental hypothermia in old people living at home and treatment before profound hypothermia has developed would seem to be the best means of reducing the mortality.

REFERENCES

1 British Medical Association, *Accidental Hypothermia in the Elderly*, *British Medical Journal*, 1964, **2**, 1255.
2 Fox, R. H., Woodward, P. M., Exton-Smith, A. N., Green, M. F. Donnison, D. V., and Wicks, M. H., *British Medical Journal*, 1973, **1**, 200.
3 Royal College of Physicians of London, *Report of Committee on Accidental Hypothermia*. London, Royal College of Physicians, 1966.
4 Fox, R. H., Woodward, P. M., Fry, A. J., Collins, J. C., and MacDonald, I. C., *Lancet*, 1971, **1**, 424.
5 Duguid, H., Simpson, R. G., and Stowers, J. M., *Lancet*, 1961, **2**, 1213.
6 Rosin, A. J., and Exton-Smith, A. N., *British Medical Journal*, 1964, **1**, 16.
7 Department of Health and Social Security, *Provision for Heating*, London, H.M.S.O., 1972.

Rehabilitation of the Elderly

BY

H. M. HODKINSON

REHABILITATION of the elderly patient—that is, helping him back to as normal a life as possible (preferably in his own home environment)—is a vital part of his hospital treatment. Unfortunately, the traditional patterns of hospital care, which were evolved at a time when most patients in hospital were young, are poorly suited to the needs of the elderly and tend to create rehabiliatation problems. Traditional care is centred on nursing in bed and the dangers of going to bed, brilliantly expounded by the late Richard Asher,[1] apply with particular force to the old. In addition, there are the dangerous institutionalizing effects of stay in hospital, the "good" patient being the one who most readily allows himself to be regimented and to accept the role of a passive yet grateful recipient of care. The important goals of self care are removed; clothes are replaced by dressing gown and slippers, so emphasizing the invalid role; and the patient is further conditioned to dependency by a plethora of professionals, whose authoritarian status is enhanced by such devices as hierarchies and uniforms. The end result is the patient who, when management decisions are put to him, says "you know best, doctor, I leave it all to you" and unquestioningly accepts being treated rather like a slow-witted child and allows things to be done for him that he can perfectly well do for himself. Here again the elderly are perhaps particularly vulnerable, being undervalued members of the community and survivors from a more authoritarian age.

A further problem is under-expectation. Elderly patients; their relatives, friends, and neighbours; and regrettably sometimes their general practitioners too tend to have an unduly pessimistic view of the likely outcome of the admission to hospital. Their long past experience of the hospital, not rarely a former "workhouse" with perhaps a former unenviable local reputation, is that the old came out of the hospital only one way—feet first. So we constantly hear such remarks as "what can you expect at my age, doctor?" from elderly patients. These prejudices need to be powerfully counteracted, for the benefits of hospital treatment stand up to comparison with those for younger age-groups[2] and most patients can be discharged home again after treatment in an active geriatric department.[3]

THE RIGHT ATMOSPHERE

It is therefore vital that an atmosphere of activity and optimism exists in the geriatric wards of the hospital. The right climate, which has such powerful effects on the expectations and progress of the individual patient, depends on many different groups: other patients, relatives, nurses, doctors, voluntary helpers, ward orderlies, porters, ministers of religion, social workers, and paramedical therapists. This very large group of individuals forms a "therapeutic community" and it is this—and not just the "rehabilitation team" of physiotherapists, occupational therapists, speech therapist, and doctors—which determines the quality of rehabilitation in the hospital ward. Good communication is needed if rehabilitation is to thrive. The ward sister, paramedical therapists, and medical staff are important group leaders, who need to create and maintain the right attitudes of enthusiasm and optimism around them; to help and direct others in the application of rehabilitation techniques; and to support and show appreciation of the value of all those forming the therapeutic community.

The establishment of an appropriate rehabilitation environment for the elderly in a ward is greatly helped by its specialized geriatric function, and this is perhaps the major justification for the separation of geriatrics from general medicine. Seeing other patients improve and go home is an undoubted encouragement to the individual patient. More active departments have an advantage here[3] and progressive patient care systems are practised in most departments, long-stay patients being transferred to other accommodation to maintain greater activity in the admission and rehabilitation wards.

NURSING STAFF ROLE

Nursing staff play a very important part. Because of their close contact with patients, relatives, and visitors it is they who can best communicate the therapeutic as opposed to custodial orientation of the department. Nursing attitudes and practice need to be adapted to the elderly. Rather than merely minister to the patient, the geriatric nurse needs to help the patient to help himself and so foster increasing independence. Firm but sympathetic re-education may be needed to modify the patient's expectations. Overprotective attitudes must be abandoned: "don't you walk on your own, you might fall" may negate all that the physiotherapist has done to build up walking skill and confidence. Nurses need to be intimately involved in the rehabilitation of the patient and so must know what stage the physiotherapist or occupational therapist has reached so as to supplement what is being done. Otherwise wily old patients often have the nurse lifting and supporting them when capable of getting up unaided and walking only with supervision by the physiotherapist, or undressing them and helping them into bed when they had dressed themselves and got in and out of bed unaided in the occupational therapy department earlier.

The elderly patient in need of rehabilitation may have a specific disability such as hemiplegia, Parkinsonism, or arthritis. More commonly, however, there is no major specific disability but the necessity to get back to normal activities after a period of illness, particularly where this has involved bed rest, which has resulting in impairment of balance, walking, and other basic skills.

In assessing the individual patient's potential for improvement full and accurate evaluation of his physical disabilities is clearly important, but it must be coupled with full consideration of mental factors and the social background. Mental factors are of paramount importance, for well-motivated patients with intact intelligence can often overcome the most daunting physical disabilities while patients with poor motivation, depression, or dementia may do badly even with fairly minor physical disabilities. Routine assessment of intellectual function by a simple orientation and memory questionnaire may be valuable in planning the patient's rehabilitation.[4] Social factors determine the specific aims of treatment—for example, whether the patient needs to be able to climb stairs, whether cooking is required, and what degree of self care is essential. Social factors may bear on motivation, with return home the desired goal for most. Others may have to accept more restricted goals, such as admission to a welfare home, and the social worker may need to help patients to adjust to such changes without losing heart. We may have to accept that the patient wants to go back to a far-from-ideal home and we may destroy his motivation if we overpersuade him to accept some seemingly more satisfactory alternative plan.

BASIC REQUIREMENTS

The basic requirements in the individual patient's rehabilitation programme will thus vary. Nevertheless, common to the majority will be the ability to walk with or without mechanical aids, to get up and down from a chair and in and out of bed, to manage the lavatory, and to dress. Stairs, cooking, and other household tasks may be needed also. The occupational therapist is concerned with determining these needs—the so-called activities of daily living (ADL) and in retraining to reach the necessary standards in the hospital ADL Department. When necessary she may arrange home modifications, clothing changes (zips or Velcro to replace difficult buttons, for example), or the provision of gadgets to simplify difficult tasks (for example, a wide variety of gadgets to enable the patient with hemiplegia to do tasks with one hand instead of two). For severely disabled patients extensive thought, re-education, and training may be needed, but more commonly patients need a check-through of ADL and brief practice to regain their confidence.

Remobilization is the principal concern of the physiotherapist. Treatment needs to start as soon as possible; otherwise strength, confidence, morale, and balance may all deteriorate rapidly—for example, rehabilitation of the stroke patient starts as soon as consciousness has returned. The patient practises rising from a chair of suitable seat height, by pushing strongly on its arms while leaning well forwards with feet kept under the front edge of the chair. If needed, help is given with hand-lifting under the axilla. Walking practice commonly uses the walking frame, which gives patients considerable support and confidence. A very simply gait pattern may be taught; the frame is advanced about 18 in (45 cm) and planted securely, the patient takes a short step with each foot, stops, and advances the frame to repeat the cycle. Even this simple regimen may call for repeated instruction of confused patients—indeed, the essentials in geriatric rehabilitation are simplicity, consistency, and repetition. Initially a helper at each side may be needed, but usually progress to walking independently in the frame is rapid. With very disabled patients one may settle for this level of activity. Otherwise progress to a stick and then no aid is typically smooth; patients do not become "addicted" to their frame if their rehabilitation is satisfactorily directed. In hemiplegics one may be obliged to use the less satisfactory tripod rather than a frame if only one hand can grip.

In supporting geriatric rehabilitation the stimulation of the patient's motivation and showing approval of success are important, and the therapist's main tool is her own personality, not complicated apparatus or techniques. Some patients, particularly during the early stages of their rehabilitation, need considerable pressure put on them by the therapist to augment their poor motivation. The successful therapist is the one who can support, encourage, and if necessary push the patient hard without alienating him and can flexibly adapt the approach used to the personality of the patient.

MAINTAINING IMPROVEMENT AT HOME

When the geriatric patient is home again, the doctor is chiefly concerned to maintain the level of activity achieved by rehabilitation. Hence it is important that all concerned should know what this level was, or the patient may slide back to an unnecessarily dependent role. Attendance at a day centre or day hospital may be a helpful stimulus. Modifications of the home may be helpful—for example, fixing handrails or providing more suitable toilet accommodation. Alternatively more suitable chairs, wheelchairs, or bath aids may be necessary. Many local authorities now employ domiciliary occupational therapists to help in such matters. Moving the bed downstairs may be a great help but should not be done without careful thought, for many old people who walk poorly on the level manage stairs very well because of the help from the stair hand-rails. In such a case bringing down the bed may encourage the invalid role and at the same time cause unnecessary major inconvenience to the other members of the family.

Though this account of rehabilitation of the elderly has emphasized the part played by hospital treatment, the general practitioner has an important part to play. He can be the most powerful influence in the re-education of the elderly and of their relatives, so that they come to have less pessimistic expectations and are aware of the potential benefits of inpatient rehabilitation. He can best do this when supported by an active geriatric service which has no waiting list. He can then help his elderly patients by early referral rather than waiting till a crisis has developed, not accepting advancing disability as an inevitable concomitant of ageing but regarding it as a diagnostic and therapeutic challenge.

REFERENCES

[1] Asher, R. A. J., *British Medical Journal*, 1947, **2**, 967.
[2] Arnold, J., and Exton-Smith, A. N., *Lancet*, 1962, **2**, 551.
[3] Hodkinson, H. M., and Jefferys, P. M., *British Medical Journal*, 1972, **4**, 536.
[4] Denham, M. J., and Jefferys, P. M., *Modern Geriatrics*, 1972, **2**, 275.

Disturbances of the Special Senses and Other Functions

BY

W. J. NICHOLSON

SENSORY deprivation is now known to be a powerful weapon in causing perceptual disturbances.[1] Maintenance of contact with reality demands stimulation from the environment, and hence it is not surprising that old people who are deaf or blind or both appear to be confused—the links of communication to a sensorium with diminishing reserve have been severed. Social isolation and loss of independence are associated with loss of the special senses. These are compelling reasons to ensure that every old person can see and hear to his or her maximum capacity.

Impairment of hearing is often due to hard plugs of wax; removal by syringing after several days softening with Cerumol ear drops is a simple procedure. If deafness persists after removing the wax it is most likely to be due to either middle ear deafness or nerve deafness. A vibrating tuning fork is applied to the vertex of the skull in the midline and the patient is asked (in writing if necessary) to indicate whether the sound is heard in midline or in either ear (Weber's test); in middle ear deafness the sound is localized in the affected ear but in nerve deafness it is localized in the normal ear. In Rinne's test the vibrating tuning fork is applied to the mastoid process, the ipsilateral ear being closed. The patient is asked to indicate when the sound ceases and the vibrating tuning fork is then placed over the ipsilateral ear. In middle ear deafness nothing can be heard, but in nerve deafness the sound can still be heard. Most patients with middle ear deafness benefit from a hearing aid but in nerve deafness do not.

Otosclerosis is the commonest cause of middle ear deafness; rarer causes are Menière's disease, acute labyrinthitis, trauma, and therapy with streptomycin or ethacrynic acid. If the ipsilateral corneal reflex is absent then a full investigation for acoustic neuroma must be made.[2]

Efforts to preserve the sight must be no less vigorous, and mere chronological age is never a contraindication to cataract extraction. Sudden loss of vision in either eye demands sudden specialist attention lest the treatable go untreated. Acute glaucoma, arteritis, internal carotid artery occlusion, and detached retina all cause sudden deterioration in vision and are treatable. Detached retina is recognized when a well-demarcated area of the retina is seen moving like a sail with a well-defined margin; often there is associated haemorrhage into the vitreous. A pale optic disc with unfilled blood vessels is seen in carotid occlusion. A profuse haemorrhagic area indicates a venous thrombosis —usually limited to one venous segment. Primary optic atrophy is recognized by the appearance of a well-defined pale disc with the attenuation of all blood vessels; treatment of the cause such as syphilis can arrest the deterioration in vision. Unilateral or asymmetrical primary optic atrophy may result from a pituitary tumour or a sphenoidal wing meningioma.

Paget's disease of the skull may compress both optic nerves, with complete blindness, and the eighth nerve, with deafness. The value of thyrocalcitonin has so far not been proved in this condition, but when the sight and hearing are threatened it may offer the possibility of preserving them.[3] Elderly people may have primary optic atrophy from toxic exposure in earlier life such as tobacco, quinine, methyl alcohol, or inorganic arsenic about which nothing can be done. Chronic glaucoma may progress to give little more than tunnel vision, so that the patient may present with a history of bumping into objects. A hemianopia is invariably associated with a hemiplegia or some other evidence of a stroke.

HEADACHE

Headache is not a feature of hypertension or space-occupying lesions in the elderly.

The headache of temporal arteritis represents an emergency because of the danger of sudden blindness[4] due to occlusion of the ophthalmic branch of the internal carotid artery. The patient with temporal arteritis may be vaguely unwell with limb pains and pyrexia; alternatively, the condition may present with sudden headache and vomiting. The ESR is always raised. Examination of the temporal or occipital arteries will show a tender swollen artery which does not pulsate. The pathological process is one of gradual arterial occlusion and therefore warrants immediate therapy with steroids (60 mg prednisolone daily). To avoid the dangers of long-term steriod therapy the affected artery should be biopsied because this minor operation seems to cause the condition to remit.

Cervical spondylosis is a common cause of occipital headache. Glaucoma may present with headache, vomiting, and photophobia; the increased intraoccular tension differentiates it from subarachnoid haemorrhage and meningitis. Headache due to arthritis of the temperomandibular joint is episodic and always worse at meal times. Sinusitis produces a headache which builds up to maximum intensity in the early afternoon and subsides towards evening; often there is an associated upper respiratory infection.

Tension headache is common and is recognized by the patient's description of "like a weight on top" or "like a band around the head"; headache associated with depression is recognized because usually there are other symptoms or signs of the condition.

FACIAL PAIN

Trigeminal neuralgia or tic doulourex has its highest incidence in elderly women, being characterized by paroxysmal sharp pain in the second or third division of the trigeminal nerve. The pain begins suddenly and usually lasts about thirty seconds: eating, talking, touching the face, or a cold wind may all precipitate an attack. Spasm of the affected side of the face may occur with closing the eye and lachrymation. There are no abnormal physical signs between attacks. The waxing and waning nature of this affliction is seen in the middle aged but it wanes less often in the old patient, who may develop a depressive illness. The introduction of carbamazepine has changed the management of trigeminal neuralgia: rarely is alcohol injection or surgical resection of the trigeminal ganglion required nowadays. The side effects of giddiness and drowsiness make it imperative to introduce carbamazepine gradually, from 100 mg once daily to a maximum dosage of 200 mg thrice daily. This drug is an anticonvulsant with the usual toxic effects of agranulocytosis and aplastic anaemia.

HERPES ZOSTER

Herpes zoster, or shingles, has its highest incidence in older patients. It is an acute virus infection involving the first sensory neurone with a papulovesicular eruption in the corresponding dermatome. A few days of pain in the dermatome often precede the appearance of the segmental rash. Dusting powder and dry dressings on the eruption are usually all that is necessary but if there is secondary infection then systemic rather than local antibiotic therapy is indicated. Zoster may affect the ophthalmic division of the fifth cranial nerve, with corneal lesions and the risk of optic neuritis; when the sight is in jeopardy urgent systemic steroid therapy is required. Rarely zoster affects the geniculate ganglion, with the pain in the ear, lower motor neurone facial paralysis, giddiness, deafness, and loss of taste in the anterior two-thirds of the tongue (Ramsay Hunt's syndrome). Most patients with herpes zoster recover without complications, the rash subsiding after seven days; however, a few develop postherpetic neuralgia, with intractable pain associated with depression. Many therapies have been tried for this condition but none seem any more effective than simple analgesics.

VERTIGO

Vertigo may be a crippling malady. The commonest cause is postural hypotension. Normally the blood pressure remains constant irrespective of the posture; this independence of posture is maintained by baroreceptor reflexes operating from the aorta and the carotid sinuses. In old age the postural change requires a longer time for baroreceptor adjustment, especially when cerebrovascular disease is present[5]; hence rapid standing up can cause momentary dizziness. Old people should get out of bed in three stages;[6] they should first sit up, they should then dangle the legs over the side of the bed, and finally stand up. That an elderly person who feels giddy has postural hypotension can easily be confirmed by recording the blood pressure lying down, sitting, and standing. Clearly only one reading taken lying down can be deceptive. Postural hypotension is a manifestation of various diseases which interrupt or slow down the baroreceptor efferent pathway, and commonly it is seen in patients who are recovering from an illness with periods of immobility—for example, a stroke or congestive cardiac failure. In these instances gradual re-education of the baroreceptor reflexes occurs with increasing mobility.

Autonomic neuropathy as in diabetes mellitus, tabes dorsalis, or acute infective polyneuropathy are rare causes of postural hypotension. Drugs often cause troublesome postural hypotension; not surprisingly adrenergic-blockers such as bethanidine do so, but many other therapeutic agents also lower the blood pressure as a side effect—for example, diuretics, barbiturates, phenothiazines, and the tricyclic antidepressants.

MENIÈRES' SYNDROME

Menière's syndrome may present for the first time in old age. The patient may have felt deaf for some time but then suddenly experiences tinnitus in one ear associated with a violent rotary sensation, vomiting, profuse sweating, and prostration. There is rotatory nystagmus maximum to the side of the affected ear, and a tremor on the finger-nose test. Prochlorperazine is useful in the acute attack, but diuretic therapy to reduce the swollen endolymphatic system is disappointing. Should the attack persist then a unilateral labyrinthectomy is indicated.

Giddiness associated with neck movement is rarely a symptom in patients with cervical spondylosis; here the atheromatous vertebral arteries are further narrowed by cervical osteophytes with resultant ischaemia of the brain stem. Other evidence of cervical spondylosis, such as wasting of the upper limb muscles or a spastic paraparesis, will be present.[7]

DROP ATTACKS

Old people often fall, but when a drop attack is the cause[8] there is a clear history that the patient fell without warning, did not lose consciousness, and had no amnesia. A patient may be standing or walking when the episode occurs; the patient rises quickly to her feet again; and there are no abnormal physical signs in the legs. Such attacks appear related to sudden failure of extensor tone in the legs but there is no evidence that vertebrobasilar insufficiency is the cause. There is no known treatment, but drop attacks wax and wane in frequency and often remit completely.

SUBDURAL HAEMATOMA

The highest incidence of subdural haematoma is in the elderly and in infants, with males predominating. Trauma is the commonest cause, but a history of this is often unobtainable, and when a good history is obtained the trauma may have been minimal. There is a recognized association with alcoholism. The diagnosis is easy if the symptoms immediately follow an injury, but this is infrequently the case; more often there is an insidious onset weeks or months after the injury with fluctuating headache, drowsiness, and confusion.[9] Focal cerebral symptoms are unusual, but when present give a clinical picture resembling a stroke. Subdural haematoma are frequently bilateral. Electroencephalography is a disappointing test in the diagnosis of subdural haematoma, being less informative than the echo ultrasound; though angiography is hazardous, it is the best investigation, showing displacement of the cerebral arteries away from the inner table of the skull.

EPILEPSY

The onset of epilepsy in the elderly usually follows a cerebrovascular accident; the seizure is grand mal in type and Jacksonian episodes are infrequent. A history of a recent stroke and the association of an upper motor neurone lesion in one or more limbs will be associated evidence. The fits can be controlled with primidone or phenytoin.

Uraemia, hypoglycaemia, and variable heart block may all provoke epileptiform seizures. In those patients with late onset epilepsy for which there is no obvious aetiology it is alway a difficult problem to balance the points for and against a full neurological investigation; however, to do so one should be influenced by the patient's biological rather than chronological age.

THE DEMENTIAS

There is wide individual variation in intellectual impairment in old age—a point appreciated fully when one sees a 95-year-old who is clear in the head attempting to converse with a confused 70-year-old. For treatment and management it is mandatory to find the aetiology of the dementia, which is not a disease in its own right but a manifestation of a disease. Dementia secondary to vascular change is always associated with lateralizing neurological signs, such as a hemiplegia or bilateral extensor plantar responses. Other evidence of vascular disease is often found—for example, coronary artery disease or peripheral vascular disease.

Senile dementia or primary neuronal dementia is not associated with neurological signs or with vascular change. Prognostically the distinction is important. Patients with arteriosclerotic dementia may live indefinitely, but those with primary neuronal dementia rarely survive for more than 18 months after the diagnosis is made. Much evidence suggests that primary neuronal dementia has a genetic basis but few patients who carry the gene survive to the age when the effects are obvious.[10]

A treatable cause of dementia is normal pressure hydrocephalus. The aetiology and incidence of this are still undetermined, but these patients improve quickly after neurosurgical shunting of the ventricular cerebrospinal fluid into the venous system.[11] [12]

CONCLUSION

Maintenance of cerebration, ambulation, sight, and hearing are essential for the quality of life and for an independent existence. The essentials depend more on the integrity of the central nervous system than on any other system.

REFERENCES

[1] Brown, J. A. C., Techniques of Persuasion, p. 246. Harmondsworth, Penguin Books, 1963.
[2] Parker, H. L., Archives of Neurology and Psychiatry, 1928, 20, 309.
[3] Woodhouse, N. J. Y., et al., Lancet, 1971, 1, 1139.
[4] Allison, R. S., The Senile Brain, p. 45. London, Arnold, 1963.
[5] Gross, M., Quarterly Journal of Medicine, 1970, 39, 485.
[6] Anderson, W. F., Practical Management of the Elderly, p. 96. Oxford, Blackwell, 1967.
[7] Brain, W. R., Northfield, D. W. C., and Wilkinson, M., Brain, 1952, 75, 187.
[8] Sheldon, J. H., British Medical Journal, 1960, 2, 1685.
[9] McKissock, W., Richardson, A., and Bloom, W. H., Lancet, 1960, 1, 1365.
[10] Isaacs, B., Introduction to Geriatrics, p. 108. London, Balliere, Tindall, and Cassell, 1965.
[11] Lancet, 1970, 2, 1074.
[12] British Medical Journal, 1973, 2, 260.

Gastrointestinal Problems in the Old—I

BY

DENNIS E. HYAMS

GASTROINTESTINAL symptoms and diseases increase with ageing, and the commonest lesions are carcinoma (of the stomach or large bowel), peptic ulceration, intestinal obstruction (herniae or diverticular disease of the colon), hiatus hernia, and gallstones. The first three of these caused most of the 20% of deaths directly due to lesions of the digestive system in McKeown's series of 1,500 necropsies in patients aged 70 or over.[1] This incidence was second only to diseases of the cardiovascular system as causes of death, and numerically only a little less. Carcinomas of the gastrointestinal system made up nearly half of the total of fatal malignant disease, and half of these were in the large bowel. Disease of the biliary tract has been said to be the commonest pathological finding requiring abdominal surgery in the aged.[2] In elderly patients with abdominal pain, Ponka et al. found that gallbladder disease was the cause in 27·5%.[3]

FUNCTIONAL CHANGES IN THE GUT

Changes have been described in the flow and composition of saliva, gastric juice, bile, and pancreatic juice; in the motility of the stomach and large bowel; in small intestinal absorption; and in large bowel flora. Associated structural changes have also been described. It is doubtful, however, whether these changes contribute significantly to gastrointestinal morbidity in old age.[4]

COMMON SYMPTOMS

Anorexia

Appetite may be reduced because of impaired sense of smell and taste, limited activity, dull food, for psychological reasons, or because of various organic disease states. About 10% of old people are housebound, which increases their vulnerability to many problems. Food may be dull or inadequate when old people find it difficult to obtain—owing to physical disabilities, lack of help, or mental confusion. Depression, isolation, loneliness, apathy, and negativism are all well-known causes of anorexia in the elderly—who are especially vulnerable after bereavement, particularly if living alone. Anorexia is seen in disease of the digestive system, notably carcinoma of the stomach, but is also a frequent symptom in physical disorders elsewhere which have secondary effects on the stomach (heart failure, anaemia, uraemia). Anorexia may also arise from their treatment (such as with digitalis, see below).

Management

Underlying causes must be identified and dealt with. Food should be attractively presented. Attempts to stimulate a poor appetite in old people by drugs, such as cyproheptadine, the old-fashioned nux vomica, or tonics such as Villescon are rarely successful. Alcohol may be more useful. Supplementary feeding (for example, with Complan) may be necessary at times to tide over a difficult period in or after an acute illness; in very weak or ill patients this may have to be given by gastric tube; rarely, parenteral feeding is required. Some very old people reject food or spit it out during feeding. Tube-feeding should be used in such cases only after careful consideration has been given to the medical and ethical aspects of the problem. Even in such cases, however, it is important to avoid dehydration.

Increased appetite in the elderly is usually psychogenic. It is rarely a feature in the elderly thyrotoxic patient.

Nausea and Vomiting

Nausea and vomiting may be due to diseases of the digestive system itself, or to diseases located primarily elsewhere. It is worth considering this latter group in more detail. Thus heart failure leads to gastric congestion and may produce anorexia, nausea, and vomiting. Cardiac infarction may also be associated with these symptoms. Digitalis intoxication may cause nausea and vomiting, though in the old it is more likely to present as an arrhythmia or a confusional state. This is an important cause of morbidity in the elderly and special care needs to be taken over the use of Lanoxin brand, which is now twice as potent on a weight-for-weight basis as formerly. Plasma digoxin assays are available in some areas and may be helpful if correlated with the clinical state, but in all cases an attempt should be made to relate digoxin dosage to renal function.

Other drugs may produce nausea and vomiting—for example, oestrogens, codeine, dihydrocodeinone, or phenformin. Metabolic disorders are another important cause, especially uraemia, diabetic ketosis, and hypercalcaemia. Labyrinthine disturbance, neurological disorders, and infections are other possible causes.

Management

The essential principle in management is to treat the underlying cause. For symptomatic treatment, antihistamines and phenothiazines have a time-honoured place as antiemetics, but are rarely without sedative side effects, which may be a nuisance in the elderly patient (who is sometimes unduly sensitive to such effects). Maxolon (metoclopramide) may be of use if this is the case.

Dysphagia

This is a common and important complaint in the old. It must *never* be regarded as functional unless the fullest possible investigation has been carried out—and even then the patient must be reviewed frequently and carefully. The difficulty in swallowing may affect solids but not liquids, and some types of solid food are easier to cope with than others. Food may stick at a consistent level, and then move on or be regurgitated, but the elderly patient's description of the level may be inaccurate. At times the initiation of the swallow reflex seems impaired, and food is chewed for long periods but finally rejected. The risk of "spillover" into the trachea is common in patients with neurologically-caused dysphagia, and they may be afraid to swallow. The alarm which dysphagia causes to an elderly patient must always be remembered: the fear of cancer will be there.

Causes of Dysphagia

Type	Position	Causes
Local	Mouth Larynx Pharynx	Tongue lesions, especially carcinoma Carcinoma Diverticulum (usually traction) Postcricoid web (Paterson-Kelly syndrome) or carcinoma Infections, abscess
	Oesophagus *Intrinsic*	Carcinoma (especially mid-level) Stricture (hiatus hernia) Spasm ("corkscrew" oesophagus) Achalasia Diverticula (traction)
	Extrinsic	Pressure (unfolded aorta—"dysphagia lusoria") Foreign body
	Stomach	Carcinoma of cardia Hiatus hernia (rolling—paraoesophageal—or sliding with ulceration or stricture)
Remote	Neurological	Disorders of brain-stem (pseudobulbar palsy, stroke, posterior inferior cerebellar artery syndrome)

Management

The primary cause must be dealt with as effectively as possible. The ethical problems of prolonged tube-feeding have been mentioned briefly above. The situation is influenced, on the one hand, by the likely prognosis and quality of life, and, on the other, by the likely mode of death—an aspect too often neglected by doctors. Neither choking nor dehydration permits death with dignity. Where a naso-gastric tube cannot be passed, a Mousseau-Barbin tube may be inserted at oesophagoscopy, to maintain a lumen in the oesophagus. Gastrostomy is not justified in the elderly—and perhaps not at any age, as it produces so much distress itself.

Change in Bowel Habit

This must always be taken seriously.

Diarrhoea

Acute diarrhoea may occur for the usual reasons (food poisoning, dietary indiscretion), but inquiry should also be made for possible abuse of purgatives. Spurious diarrhoea, due to faecal impaction (see below), is common in old people.

Chronic diarrhoea raises the suspicion of carcinoma of the colon or rectum, but may also be due to other diseases of the gastrointestinal tract, especially diverticular disease of the colon, ulcerative coloproctitis, or commonly faecal impaction. Diarrhoea may be due to steatorrhoea, possibly after an earlier partial gastrectomy, or due to abuse of pur-gatives.

Systemic disorders associated with diarrhoea include uraemia, diabetes, thyrotoxicosis, and liver disease. Psychogenic causes may occur in old age, as in younger persons.

Old people with diarrhoea may develop faecal incontinence due to the urgency of the desire to defaecate, the fluid or semi-formed stool, and possibly impaired mobility, a too-distant lavatory, and occasionally laxity or weakness of the anal sphincter.

Faecal Incontinence

The causes of faecal incontinence may be local or distant. Of local causes, diarrhoea is the commonest, but rectal prolapse or prolapsed haemorrhoids may be present. Rarely is faecal incontinence due to simply weakness of laxity of the sphincter. Distant causes include brain damage or dementia, leading to lack of cortical inhibition, but this cause is less common than a local cause—in contrast to urinary incontinence, where the converse applies. Spinal cord lesions are rare causes of faecal incontinence in the old.

Faecal incontinence can be the final straw which breaks down attempts to nurse an old person at home; by earning for him the erron-eous label of "senile" or "mental" it may lead to misplacement of the patient in a mental hospital.

Constipation

Many old people are constipated, and even more are convinced that they are, since preoccupation with the bowels is common in old age. The importance of constipation is that it may lead to severe complications. Constipation is best thought of not in terms of transit-time through the gut, which is slowed in old age[5][6] without necessarily causing symptoms, but rather the type of faeces produced—that is, hard and dry.

About half the elderly people studied in various surveys take laxatives, often unnecessarily.

Causes: Primary causes are slow transit-time (especially in bedfast patients); incomplete enptying (poor muscle tone, unsatisfactory toilet arrangements, laziness, mental confusion, or dementia); diminished awareness of a loaded or overloaded rectum; neglect of the call to defaecate; low-bulk diet (ignorance, cost, poor dentition); and inadequate fluid (sometimes due to fear of urinary difficulties).

Secondary causes of constipation may be gastrointestinal or otherwise. Diverticular disease of the colon and carcinoma of the colon or rectum must be considered. Anorectal lesions such as fissures, haemorrhoids, or pectenosis[7] may contribute.

Other important causes include drugs (codcine and dihydrocodeine, morphine, iron, aluminium compounds, calcium salts, and anticholinergics), hypothyroidism, and mental disorders.

Combined causes may also be present. As usual in the elderly, there may be several factors operating to produce the disability Wilkins has illustrated the vicious circles which may develop (fig.).[8]

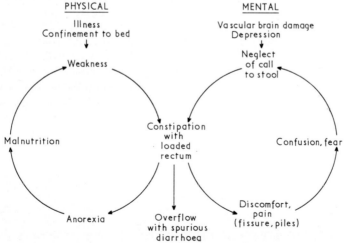

Vicious Circles of Constipation in the Elderly[8]

Complications: The main complication is faecal impaction. Faecal retention plus absorption of fluid in the large bowel leads to hardening of faeces, which are packed together by peristaltic waves and lubricated by excess secretion of mucus. The impaction over-distends the rectum; but very occasionally it may occur higher in the colon while the rectum remains empty. Sometimes impaction of a great mass of soft faeces occurs in weak patients.

Faecal impaction may lead to:

(1) *Faecal incontinence.* Impacted faeces act as a ball-valve and more liquid stool at a higher level leaks around the faecel mass. Stretching of the anal ring is corrected only when the rectum is cleared; until then the "spurious diarrhoea" will continue.

(2) *Intestinal obstruction.* This may have a high mortality or may lead to unnecessary surgical intervention.

(3) *Mental disturbances.* Restlessness and confusion may be due to faecal impaction. This might be termed the "recto-cephalic reflex". It is worth remembering this simple mechanism when dealing with disturbed or restless old people; it could save many an unwarranted admission to hospital. Sedation of the patient without a preliminary rectal examination is poor medical practice.

(4) *Retention of urine.* This may be associated with overflow urinary incontinence, possibly due to pressure of the distended rectum on the bladder neck.

(5) *Rectal bleeding.* This may occur owing to the ulceration of the mucosa; the presence of a neoplasm must be excluded.

Other gastrointestinal effects may occur with constipation—for example, megacolon, with an atonic colon, or volvulus of the colon, producing intestinal obstruction. Gross gaseous distension of the bowel may produce angina pectoris and electrocardiographic changes.

Another important complication of constipation results from straining. Adverse effects of straining have been clearly demonstrated on the coronary, cerebral, and peripheral arterial circulation. In the elderly with cerebrovascular disease transient ischaemic attacks may occur; in those with impaired baroreceptor reflexes and a tendency to postural hypotension, the Valsalva manoeuvre is produced by straining at stool and the patient may develop syncope. This mechanism may account for the not infrequent history of finding the patient on the lavatory floor.

Symptoms of hiatus hernia may be aggravated by the rise in intra-abdominal pressure on straining.

Management

Proper management of diarrhoea is impossible without a rectal examination. The underlying cause must be treated as far as possible.

For symptomatic treatment, in acute cases, food should be withheld for up to 24 hours, but fluids must be given liberally to avoid dehydration. Kaolin or activated attapulgite are available in various preparations, sometimes combined with opiates or antibiotics. They are useful for relieving symptoms but should only be used when the cause of the diarrhoea has been diagnosed with reasonable certainty. Stool cultures should be taken before using antibiotics; rectal swabs are far less reliable. In the elderly, care should be taken about the use of these medicines; it is bad clinical practice to give kaolin mixtures to patients with diarrhoea which is spurious and secondary to faecal impaction. Injudicious use of opiates may mask the diagnosis of important abdominal pathology. Lomotil is useful to reduce transit time in the intestine. Codeine phosphate tablets may also be used but may encourage vomiting. Hydrophilic bulking agents such as Metamucil, Isogel, or Celevac—while mainly of use in the treatment of constipation—may also be of value in diarrhoea if taken with jam rather than water. They then absorb water from the stool and improve its consistence. This is of particular value in helping to regulate the functioning of a colostomy.

Similar considerations apply in the management of chronic diarrhoea. Accurate diagnosis is essential. Particular attention should be paid to fluid and electrolyte (especially potassium) balance.

In the management of constipation the underlying causes must also be treated on their merits. In general management, reassurance and explanation will help if habits need re-training: physicial activity, fluid intake, and the amount of bulk in the diet require attention. Some old people are helped by a glass or hot water first thing in the morning as a regular habit. Toilet arrangements may require revision. While low lavatory seats are difficult for the elderly to cope with, some degree of squatting aids defaecation; excessive zeal in raising the level of the seat may actually hinder efficient defaecation. (Nevertheless, polyethylene seat raises are valuable to many arthritic old people.)

Laxatives: There are three main types of laxatives. Firstly, the bulking agents. Many people (old and young) live on diets low in fibre content, which produce small, hard, and infrequent stools. Bulking agents are bland and absorb water, increasing volume of the stool. This is the most physiological way of dealing with constipation and diverticular disease of the colon.

Unprocessed bran is an ideal additive to the diet in such cases—and in their prevention. It may be sprinkled on cereals or other foodstuffs. Probably most old people would benefit from its regular consumption, but its high phytic acid content might impair calcium absorption in subjects with latent or overt vitamin D deficiency—and there is increasing evidence that this might be commoner in the elderly than previously thought. Other hydrophilic agents in this category include semi-synthetic cellose ethers (Celevac, Cellucon, and Cologel), and mucilaginous substances (Metamucil, Isogel, and Normacol). These agents should be taken with abundant liquids to avoid the potential hazard of intestinal obstruction from bolus formation, especially when intestinal motility is reduced or if there is intestinal disease.

The second type of laxatives are the stimulant ones. The anthracene laxatives are best represented by senna, available in standardized form as Senokot. Its main effect is on the transverse and distal colon, so that stools are likely to be formed, and fluid and electrolyte disturbances are unlikely.

Bisacodyl (Dulcolax) is a contact laxative and more likely than Senokot to produce liquid stools and (in the elderly) the risk of faecal incontinence; it is also more likely to cause severe griping. Phenolphthalein has no place in modern therapeutics.

The other stimulant laxatives, including irritants like colocynth, jalap, podophyllum, aloes (all contained in vegetable laxative tablets), and croton-oil, have no place in modern management of constipation at any age.

Thirdly, the osmotic laxatives, or "salts"—soluble sulphates, phosphates or tartrates of sodium, potassium or magnesium—act by the osmotic effect of their ions retaining large volumes of fluid throughout the bowel. The disturbance to normal gut physiology is considerable, the stools are loose, and fluid and electrolyte disturbance likely. These agents are best kept for special indications only (for example, food-poisoning). Lactulose acts only when acted on by colonic bacteria; it may cause gaseous distension, but this is usually transient. It is useful to clear the bowel and lower the faecal pH as methods of combating ammonia intoxication in chronic portal-systemic encephalopathy,[9] and it has been recommended for the prevention and treatment of colonic retention of barium after a barium meal.[10]

Stool Softeners: Dioctylsodium sulphosuccinate (DOS) (Di-octyl Forte, Coprola) and poloxalkols are surface-active "wetting" agents, which are said to penetrate hard stools and to help soften them. The formation of hard stools is said to be prevented during the administration of these drugs. They are popular in geriatric practice, but it is only fair to point out that the possible effects (especially the long-term ones) of the consumption of detergents are not yet fully known. In animals they have been shown to cause changes in gut physiology.

Combinations of these agents with stimulant laxatives (for example, Dulcodos, bisacodyl plus DOS; Dorbanex, danthron plus poloxalkols) have been found useful in geriatric patients, but, again, some caution it required, since other combinations of this type have had adverse effects in large doses or in chronic usage.

Liquid paraffin, once thought harmless, has now earned itself a bad name. It may impair absorption of fat-soluble vitamins, leak from the anus, be aspirated into the lungs to cause lipoid pneumonia, and be absorbed (especially when given in emulsion form) and be deposited in body tissue. These risks are greater in the elderly, and its use should be avoided—at least as a regular habit.

Rectal Evacuation: Suppositories of glycerine or bisacodyl are sometimes helpful. The latter may cause local discomfort. Enemas should be small-volume solutions: oil for softening and saline for evacuation. Disposable hypertonic saline enemas are convenient, gentle, and reasonably effective. Soap should never be used in enemas.

Manual Removal of Faeces: This may be required in the initial treatment of faecal impaction: oral laxatives cannot be expected to clear the bowel when the lower end is plugged so effectively with accumulated faeces. Suppositories and enemas may also fail in this situation, although a small-volume enema should be tried as the first step, and this may be repeated daily, its efficacy being judged by repeated digital examinations. With soft faecal impaction bisacodyl supporitories may also be successful: one should be used high up in the rectum and repeated once if there has been no result after two hours.

Large volume washouts with saline may be needed to clear the lower bowel if impaction is high above the rectum.

In the management of faecal incontinence, since most cases are due to spurious diarrhoea associated with faecal impaction, treatment of the latter will deal with the incontinence. For the neurogenic types of faecal incontinence, a regimen of Mist. kaolin et morph, 15 ml every morning, alternating with Senokot 1-2 tablets every night has been advocated by Jarrett and Exton-Smith.[11] In such cases it is essential to exclude the presence of faecal impaction.

REFERENCES

[1] McKeown, F., *Pathology of the Aged*. Butterworth, London, 1965.
[2] Strohl, E. L., Diffenbaugh, W. G., and Anderson, R. E., *Geriatrics*, 1964, **19**, 275.
[3] Ponka, J. L., Welborn, J. K., and Brush, B. E., *Journal of the American Geriatrics Society*, 1963, **11**, 993.
[4] Hyams, D. E., *Modern Geriatrics*, 1973, **3**, 352.
[5] Hyams, D. E., *Gerontologia Clinica*, 1964, **6**, 193.
[6] Brocklehurst, J. C., and Kahn, M. Y., *Gerontologia Clinica*, 1969, **11**, 293.
[7] Exton-Smith, A. N., in *Management of Constipation*, p. 156. Avery-Jones, F., and Godding, E. W., Blackwell Scientific Publications, Oxford, 1972.
[8] Wilkins, E. G., *Postgraduate Medical Journal*, 1968, **44**, 728.
[9] Elkington, S. G., *Gut*, 1970, **11**, 1043.
[10] Prout, B. J., Datta, S. B., and Wilson, T. S., *British Medical Journal*, 1972, **4**, 530.
[11] Jarrett, A. S., and Exton-Smith, A. N., *Lancet*, 1960, **1**, 925.

Gastrointestinal Problems in the Old—II

BY

DENNIS E. HYAMS

ACUTE ABDOMEN

THE acute abdomen often causes considerable problems in elderly patients. Its presentation may be atypical, its course more stormy with later diagnosis and a much greater likelihood of complications— especially at and after surgery.

Old people are often less able to cope with their illness than are younger patients, so that early diagnosis becomes of major importance; yet these are often the very patients who are diagnosed late because of difficulties in communication, few or atypical symptoms, absence of "classical" physical signs, and difficulty in physical examination due to associated degenerative or disease processes. Pain may be absent or unimpressive and the description of its type and site is often vague. Abdominal rigidity, and even guarding, may be absent where it would certainly have been present in earlier years, and in such patients the presence or absence of gut sounds can become a most important physical sign, the situation being in many ways analogous to the acute abdomen developing in a patient being treated with steroids.

Complications occur frequently: thus, complications of acute appendicitis are found at operation five times more often in the old than in younger patients. Peritonitis from whatever cause is less effectively kept localized in elderly patients. The mortality of major operations is increased several-fold, especially if the operation is performed as an emergency. The mortality rate increases in the elderly as age advances.

It is a good general rule to admit to hospital elderly people with severe abdominal pain, even if there are no physical signs. It must be remembered that many medical causes of acute abdominal pain may occur in the elderly, including acute pancreatitis, diabetic ketosis, tabes dorsalis, Addison's disease, hypercalcaemia, haemochromatosis, or porphyria. Furthermore, abdominal pain may be due to extra-abdominal disease—for example, pleurisy, spondylosis, zoster, etc.— and these are common in old people. For an excellent review of the acute abdomen in the elderly, see Charlesworth.[1]

SOME INDIVIDUAL CONDITIONS
Diverticular Disease
Small Intestine

Duodenal diverticula are common, second only to colonic. They

146

occur in about 10% of people after 55 years of age. They have for long been regarded as being of little or no clinical significance unless complications develop; but Clark[2] has reviewed the literature, adding 15 cases of his own, and has emphasized that duodenal diverticular disease may be associated with altered bowel flora, producing a form of stagnant loop syndrome with malabsorption and deficiency states analogous to those found with jejunal diverticulosis. The actual deficiencies seem to differ in prevalence from those in the jejunal variety, so that iron, folate, and vitamin B_{12} deficiency were seen in that order of frequency (the reverse of the jejunal pattern); this may be because the altered bowel flora in duodenal cases are localized to the upper small intestine.

Colon

Colonic diverticula develop in middle and later life, especially in the obese and the constipated. They occur in one in three persons over 60. The diverticula are the result of a disturbance of colonic motility, often with hypertrophied smooth muscle, tending to produce high intraluminal pressures in the colon. Fibre-deficient diets are associated with long intestinal transit times and small infrequent stools. Such diets, with abundant refined carbohydrate encouraging fermentation in the intestine, also lead to abnormal increases of pressure in the bowel, and are important factors in the pathogenesis of diverticulosis coli.[3]

It is difficult to differentiate diverticulosis from diverticulitis clinically, and often radiologically.[4] Three clinical patterns may be recognized. Firstly, most cases are asymptomatic. Secondly, symptoms may arise in uncomplicated cases and consist of abdominal discomfort, pain in the left iliac fossa, and constipation or diarrhoea. Thirdly, in complicated diverticular disease, pain, tenderness, fever, and bleeding per rectum may occur. There may be a mass in the left side of the abdomen, and bladder involvement is occasionally seen. A pericolic abscess may form and may perforate. It is worth remembering that diverticular disease of the colon has been called "the great imitator".

Treatment has traditionally been with a low-residue diet, but Painter[5] showed that unprocessed bran was effective in relieving symptoms. It is cheap and easily taken. Daily doses of 2–12 g (1–6 teaspoonful) have been recommended, and should be continued throughout life, even in asymptomatic cases, except when complications are present. Acute symptoms still call for a low-residue diet, and drugs may be required—for example, antibiotics if infection is diagnosed, anticholinergic drugs for pain (but they may aggravate constipation), or faecal softeners to avoid obstructive episodes. Sublaxative doses of Senokot have been shown to be spasmolytic and might prove to have a place in management. Drugs to avoid are morphine, neostigmine, and the hypnotic glutethimide (which has been reported to cause smooth muscle spasm). Surgery may be needed in complicated cases.

Inflammatory Disease of the Large Bowel

In the differential diagnoses of a patient with diarrhoea, abdominal pain, change of bowel habit, and rectal bleeding, it is worth considering inflammatory conditions such as Crohn's disease and ulcerative coloproctitis. Though much rarer than carcinoma or diverticular disease, they have important differences in management and in therapeutic possibilities.

Crohn's Disease

In the elderly Crohn's disease tends to affect the distal colon and rectum, and may present at first like diverticular disease; however, persistence of modest bleeding from the rectum should suggest Crohn's rather than diverticulitis, where rectal bleeding is more likely to be intermittent and severe. Local fistulae or extraintestinal complications suggest inflammatory disease rather than diverticular disease. While the two conditions may co-exist, it is important to recognize Crohn's disease when it is present. Management calls for steroid therapy: surgical intervention often leads to complications.

Ulcerative Coloproctitis

Ulcerative coloproctitis may appear for the first time in the elderly, and is then often more persistent and with a worse prognosis than in younger subjects. Diagnosis is confirmed by endoscopy and biopsy. Management is along the usual lines, including steroid and sulphasalazine therapy.

Carcinoma of the Large Bowel

Carcinoma of the large bowel is mainly a disease of late middle and old age. Half of them are in the distal colon; and over one-third of these present with complete intestinal obstruction. Recent change of bowel habit is an important symptom; there may be passage of mucus or blood per rectum. The importance of routine rectal examination in elderly patients cannot be over-emphasized.

Bleeding is usually occult and the patient may present with iron-deficiency anaemia. This is common in old age, and its most usual cause is gastrointestinal blood loss. Haemorrhoids may be secondary to a carcinoma higher up. Proctoscopy and sigmoidoscopy should precede a request for barium enema. The latter is unlikely to be of help unless there are clinical features pointing fairly clearly to the large cut (for example, bleeding, an abdominal mass or suggestive sigmoidoscopic findings).

Intestinal Obstruction

Intestinal obstruction may be mechanical or paralytic (adynamic). The former is usually a surgical problem—the obstruction may occur in the small gut (hernia, adhesions) or large gut (carcinoma of distal colon, diverticular disease or volvulus of the colon), but the big exception is faecal impaction—easily diagnosable and amenable to medical treatment.

Adynamic obstruction is seen in mesenteric vascular occlusion, ruptured aneurysm of the abdominal aorta, acute pancreatitis, and various other causes of peritonitis.

Gastrointestinal Bleeding

Haematemesis and melaena may occur from peptic ulcer, with or without ingestion of drugs (such as aspirin, steroids, phenylbutazone, or idomethacin). Haematemesis may also—though far lass often— occur from hiatus hernia, oesophageal varices, the Mallory-Weiss syndrome, a gastric neoplasm, or a blood dyscrasia. Appreciable rectal bleeding is usually due to diverticular disease of the colon. Occult gastrointestinal bleeding may present as iron-deficiency anaemia: such patients require serial consecutive faecal occult blood tests.

Ischaemia of the Intestine

Three syndromes of intestinal ischaemia are described.

Acute Mesenteric Vascular Occlusion

Acute mesenteric vascular occlusion (arterial or venous) produces the dramatic picture of mesenteric infarction:[6] acute abdominal pain, vomiting, and diarrhoea (perhaps blood-stained), distension with little guarding, loss of gut sounds, and shock. Pre-existing cardiac disease is common and may predispose to intestinal infarction without actual obstruction of the mesenteric vessels; arterial embolism or thrombosis are the commonest lesions, however, the former usually being associated with atrial fibrillation. The prognosis is poor; massive resection of intestine gives poor results—a high mortality, or nutritional problems if the patient survives. A direct attack on the artery is more hopeful, possibly with an arterial anastomotic procedure in addition (for example, to the right common iliac artery).

Chronic Intestinal Ischaemia

Chronic intestinal ischaemia may produce either intestinal angina or ischaemic colitis.

Intestinal angina[7] present characteristically with periumbilical pain soon after meals, unrelieved by alkalis; the severity of the pain is related to the size of the meal, so that meals get smaller and weight loss appears. There may be diarrhoea. A bruit may be heard in the epigastrium, but few other signs are found. Barium studies are negative but aortography—with coeliac axis or superior mesenteric angiography or both—will show the arterial lesions.

Ischaemic colitis results from more distal obstruction in mesenteric vessels; in fact, both small and large gut may be affected, and the lesions are segmental. It is worth considering this diagnosis in the elderly with chronic diarrhoea which is not due to a more obvious cause. Barium enema may help but again the diagnosis is best made by aortography. Some cases heal but strictures may have developed. Conservative treatment is recommended if the diagnosis is certain (carcinoma being excluded, of course), unless complications such as spreading peritonitis ensue.[8]

Droller[9] reported 13 cases of atheromatous disease of the vessels supply the gut in 1,700 geriatric patients admitted consecutively to his department in Leeds.

Appendicitis

Though the clinical features of appendicitis are similar to those at younger ages, complications are found five times as often at operation. Early diagnosis is thus of extreme importance.

Peptic Ulceration

Peptic ulcer is common in the elderly: in women it is nearly always gastric; in men the duodenal/gastric ratio of 4:1 (seen at earlier ages) is maintained. The former teaching that large gastric ulcers are probably malignant is no longer acceptable in the elderly, who may develop giant gastric ulcers which are benign and may heal rapidly. On the other hand, the recurrence rate is high, and the risk of haemorrhage is real,[10] so that surgical intervention may become necessary. Acute gastric erosions may be due to drugs—especially aspirin which may be taken for condition such as arthritis.

The history of peptic ulcer in the elderly may be typical, but is often atypical and may be very short. A barium meal is often essential for the diagnosis to be made. The possibility of malignancy may be suggested—or perhaps cannot be excluded—by the results of the barium meal, and a fibreoscopy is then sometimes of value. It is important to establish an accurate diagnosis since management (as always) depends on this.

Treatment for the elderly does not include bed rest or strict dietary regimens: the former is unwise and the latter usually impracticable.

It is important to avoid smoking but this may be difficult for some old people. Alkalis and cholinergic drugs may be used with care. Carbenoxolone is to be avoided as it is apt to produce troublesome hypokalaemia in the elderly, especially those on diuretics or with liver dysfunction; there is also the possibility of salt and water retention, heart failure, and the need for further diuretic therapy. Some of the liquorice preparations such as Caved-S and Ulcedal claim to have reduced such side effects. A newer introduction for peptic ulcer is De-Nol, a chelated bismuth compound, which is said to protect the ulcer site and to promote healing of both gastric and duodenal ulcers. It is used without severe restrictions as to diet, smoking, etc., any is reported not to disturb electrolyte balance. Other new drugs of some promise include Gefarnil (gefarnate), and antipepsins or carrageenins.

Complications call for the usual prompt measures. The elderly do not tolerate haemorrhage well, especially upper gastrointestinal bleeding. Perforation may be clinically remarkably silent in old people.

Carcinoma of the Stomach

The incidence of stomach cancer increases with ageing, and is higher in association with pernicious anaemia than would be expected by chance. It is often diagnosed late owing to the insidious onset of anorexia and weight loss, and should be suspected when investigating any anaemia. The results of faecal occult blood tests, barium meal and, if indicated, fibreoscopy, will help towards the diagnosis. Exfoliative cytology may be valuable, but gastric acid studies are less valuable in the old, though if free acid is present this diagnosis is less likely.

Liver and Gall-Bladder

Structural and functional changes are slight and have been reviewed by Hyams.[11]

Jaundice

The assessment and management of jaundice in the elderly are essentially as in younger patients. The diagnosis in the old nearly always lies between gallstones, drug administration, and obstruction by neoplasm; but it is worth remembering that the commonest cause of jaundice in the elderly with congestive cardiac failure is pulmonary infarction—the increased pigment derived from the liberated haemoglobin in the infarct overloads the anoxic liver cells.

Obstructive jaundice is commoner than hepatocellular jaundice, and extrahepatic obstruction (due to neoplasm or gallstones) is commoner than intrahepatic (cholestasis, usually drug-induced). The commonest cause is neoplasm, usually carcinoma of the head of the pancreas, but sometimes metastatic neoplastic deposits in the liver or in lymph nodes at the porta hepatis. Primary carcinomas of the gallbladder and bile ducts, or of the liver itself, are rare.

Calculus obstruction to the common bile duct may be a painless illness in the elderly. Since pain, and even a fluctuating depth of jaundice, may occur in malignant cases, differential diagnosis can be difficult. It is important to avoid undue delay in establishing the diagnosis since the mortality may then rise sharply. It is recommended that if the diagnosis has not been established within six weeks of the onset of jaundice in an old person, laparotomy should be performed.

Hepatitis and Cirrhosis

Hepatitis is not common, but has a graver prognosis in old age than in younger patients. It may be difficult to diagnose and even lead to unnecessary laparotomy if it causes obstructive jaundice. Serum hepatitis is insidious in onset and affects older and iller patients than infectious hepatitis. The latter, however, tends to take on a more virulent character in the old than in the young.

Cirrhosis is not rare, but may be clinically latent. It is usually cryptogenic in old age. Primary biliary cirrhosis is sometimes seen in elderly women, who present with pruritus and, later, jaundice, malabsorption, pigmentation, xanthomata, clubbing, and hepato-(spleno-)megaly.

Haemochromatosis is occasionally seen in the elderly, and may be associated with polyarthritis.

Drugs

Drugs may adversely affect the liver, and may cause hepatic necrosis, fatty liver, a hepatitis-like reaction, or intrahepatic cholestatis. The latter may sometimes be due to hypersensitivity.

The table sets out various causes and categories of liver injury, and gives examples relevant to elderly patients. In geriatric practice, the main drugs implicated are: phenothiazines (especially chlorpromazine), antidepressants, oral hypoglycaemic agents, antirheumatic drugs, antituberculous drugs, sulphonamides, diuretics, antithyroid drugs, anticonvulsants, dichloralphenazone, and oral anabolic agents. In regard to the last group, elderly patients requiring anabolic drugs should receive injections of, say, Deca-Durabolin intramuscularly every three weeks, rather than oral agents.

Gallstones

The incidence of gallstones increases with advancing age, especially in women. Symptoms are due to complications, which develop more often in the elderly, who then fare less well than younger patients. Apart from diagnostic difficulties, surgery under non-elective conditions carries a relatively high mortality.

The commonest problem is probably the silent gallstone(s). Here, despite the risks of complications, most authors advocate a conservative

Toxic Liver Injury

Mechanism	Examples	
	Drugs	Other Agents
Hepatic necrosis	Halogenated hydro-carbons Heavy metals Cytotoxic drugs Intravenous tetracycline Overdose of iron or paracetamol	DDT (dicophane) Paraquat Benzene derivatives Amanita mushrooms Irradiation Burns Hyperpyrexia
Fatty liver	Alcohol	Various organic and inorganic chemicals Irradiation Other diseases (ulcerative colitis, diabetes, anaemia)
Hepatitis-like reaction	Antidepressants Anticonvulsants Antituberculous drugs Antirheumatic drugs Halothane	
Intrahepatic cholestatis due to hypersensitivity	Chlorpromazine Antidepressants Oral hypoglycaemic agents Benzodiazepines Thiazides Phenylbutazone Antithyroid drugs Sulphonamides	
Intrahepatic cholestasis without hypersensitivity	Methyltestosterone Oral anabolic agents	
Mixed	Antituberculous drugs Sulphonamides Oral antidiabetic agents Methyldopa Erythromycin estolate	

approach after the age of 60 years. A most exciting development is the current research on the dissolution of gallstones by oral administration of chenodeoxycholic acid.[12] [13]

Cholecystitis

Cholecystitis is usually associated with gallstones. Acute attacks may mimic other abdominal emergencies, or myocardial infarction or pleurisy. Treatment is by antibiotics and supportive therapy. Rifamide is an antibiotic which is concentrated in bile, and may be valuable; otherwise a bactericidal broad-spectrum antibiotic such as ampicillin or cephaloridine should be used. Erythromycin estolate should be avoided, and so must morphine. Complications include gangrene, perforation, or empyema of the gallbladder, and are more likely in the elderly.

British surgeons tend to be cautious about cholecystectomy soon after acute cholecystitis, but American surgeons favour intervention early after the acute stage—though the mortality still appears rather high.

Chronic cholecystitis is usually associated with gallstones, and is then the commonest disease of the biliary system. Symptoms are vague and the onset usually insidious: "flatulent dyspepsia", especially after fatty food; nausea and vomiting; discomfort in the right hypochondrium (or right scapula or shoulder). There may be tenderness over the gallbladder and a positive Murphy's sign. The picture is often atypical, and must be distinguished from hiatus hernia and peptic ulcer, colonic disorders, and urinary infections.

Oral cholecystography is often remarkably unhelpful in the elderly. Treatment may be medical and is then symptomatic, with weight reduction and restriction of fat intake; but the definitive treatment if stones are present is cholecystectomy.

REFERENCES

[1] Charlesworth, D., *Practitioner*, 1972, **209**, 178.
[2] Clark, A. N. G., *Age and Ageing*, 1972, **1**, 14.
[3] Painter, N. D., and Burkitt, D. P., *British Medical Journal*, 1971, **2**, 450.
[4] Parks, T. G., Connell, A. M., Gough, A. D., and Cole, J. O. Y., *British Medical Journal*, 1970, **1**, 136.
[5] Painter, N. S., *British Medical Journal*, 1971, **2**, 156.
[6] Jackson, B. B., *Occlusion of the Superior Mesenteric Artery*. Thomas, Springfield, Illinois, 1963.
[7] Dick, A. P., Graff, R., Gregg, D. McG., Peters, N., and Sarner, M. *Gut*, 1967, **8**, 206.
[8] Marcuson, R. W., and Farman, J. A., *Proceedings of the Royal Society of Medicine*, 1971, **64**, 1080.
[9] Droller, H., *Age and Ageing*, 1972, **1**, 162.
[10] Strange, S. L., *Gerontologia Clinica*, 1963, **5**, 171.

[11] Hyams, D. E., *Diseases of the liver and biliary system. Textbook of Geriatric Medicine and Gerontology.* J. C. Brocklehurst. Churchill Livingstone, Edinburgh and London, 1973.
[12] Danzinger, R. G., Hofmann, A. F., Schoenfield, L. J., and Thistle, J. L., *New England Journal of Medicine*, 1972, **286**, 1.
[13] Bell, G. D., Whitney, B., and Dowling, R. H., *Lancet*, 1972, **2**, 1213.

Geriatric Orthopaedics

BY

M. B. DEVAS

IN good health the aged have to face many problems in any society; to them illness comes as a catastrophe which can take away their independence. Because of this, geriatric orthopaedics has become a most stimulating and rewarding subject, which makes great demands on both medical and surgical skills as well as on enthusiastic teamwork if the problems posed by each patient are to be solved and independence to be regained.

The principles of geriatric medicine and surgery are the same as at any other age but they have to be applied with the utmost vigour from the moment of admission to the ultimate discharge from outpatients (so-called "total care".) The circumstances in which the patient lives, financial problems, the surgical condition, the concomitant medical afflictions, how rehabilitation and the social services can best be used, nursing care and, most important, the morale of the patient all have to be carefully considered. It must be remembered that in the elderly loss of function means loss of independence.

The most important physical sign in geriatric orthopaedics is to see the patient walk. The next most important is to see that the patient can undertake the ordinary activities of daily living. Hence all treatment must be aimed at the restoration of both as quickly as possible. The old person invariably has many other ailments besides that which has caused his admission to hospital, especially when the latter is caused by a fracture. Because of this treatment is best managed by a team based on a special geriatric orthopaedic unit, which is described below, to which the more enfeebled patient may be transferred as soon as possible after the necessary operation has been done.

There are two main divisions of surgical treatment: the emergency repair of a fracture, and the elective orthopaedic operation. In each, however, the same aim applies—namely, the quick return to independence.

Bed rest in the elderly is bad for many reasons, the most important being the difficulty in learning to walk again; this has to be taught to a patient after prolonged decubitus. Secondly, the activities of daily living, such as dressing and toilet, become blurred in the mind of the very old, particularly in the presence of slight confusion. Thirdly, there are various medical contraindications to bed rest; although in the immediate management of the patient they are less important, they include the increase in osteoporosis; the danger of respiratory, genitourinary, and other intercurrent infections; the liability to develop postural hypotension; and the lowering of morale of both patient and relatives. For these reasons, the best surgical procedure on an old patient is one so designed that walking can start at once. In the treatment of fractures no operation should be done that leaves the patient in bed suffering not only from the effects of the broken bone but also from those of the operation. Ideally the latter should deal curatively with the fracture, leaving the patient only to recover from an operation, which is always well tolerated in the elderly. Finally, the surgical procedure must never be considered to be the whole treatment but merely an incident in the general rehabilitation of the patient.

HIP FRACTURES

The fracture near the hip is the commonest emergency and one which can cause serious difficulties. It exemplifies the problems of management, treatment, and rehabilitation of all geriatric surgical conditions. An outline of the care of this condition will give a full understanding not only of the solution to the problem but of the philosophy needed in orthopaedics in the elderly.

Ideally in the home the family doctor, knowing his hospital, will reassure the patient that the broken hip will soon be mended and that three weeks will be ample time in which to get well and to return home; the sooner this message is understood by the patient and those around her, the better the morale.

On admission to hospital the patient is investigated by the radiology department and the clinical laboratory, with particular emphasis on the nature of the fracture, and the blood haemoglobin content, blood group, and blood urea level. Heart failure and diabetes are excluded and, if the patient is in pain, a splint is put on with a non-adhesive skin traction. Except for a few patients with unstable diabetes and untreated heart failure (in whom operation is delayed for a day or so while the condition is being stabilized), the patient is prepared for the operation, which should be done within twenty-four hours.

Before the operation the dehydrated patient is given fluids intravenously. At operation it is necessary to give blood freely; packed cells are of value to avoid overloading the circulation in very anaemic patients. An antibiotic is given routinely to cover the operation; streptomycin is to be avoided in the elderly especially if there is any form of renal failure.

Anaesthesia

There is no contraindication to a geriatric patient receiving either general or hypotensive anaesthesia, each of which materially benefits both patient and surgeon. In general, apart from untreated diabetes or heart failure, to delay operation "to improve the patient" because of other ailments has the reverse effect: once the fracture has been treated surgically movement is no longer so painful or so difficult, recovery is speedier, and walking can start.

Operation and After Care

The fractures near the hip may be divided into those of the femoral neck and those of the trochanteric region. The latter can be fixed firmly and safely by a pin-and-plate operation, which, adequately performed, allows the patient to weight bear the next day. The fracture of the femoral neck should also present no problem, though controversy still exists over the best method of treatment. Replacement of the femoral head by a Thompson type of prosthesis cemented into place gives rise to fewer problems and promotes a faster rehabilitation than does internal fixation. The wound is closed in layers with one or two suction drains. An air-permeable adhesive dressing covers the incision. The patient walks the next day. This operation, properly done, has few complications—among which dislocation of the prosthesis is conspicuously absent. Also, because a lateral approach is used, which is not near the perineum, any incontinence does not contaminate the wound; not being posterior, the approach allows the patient to lie or sit comfortably; and because it is not anterior, flexion of the hip does not cause much movement of the sutured skin edges. These points also apply to the pin and plate, which is also done through a similar approach.

After the operation pethidine or morphine are given adequately to control pain. The antibiotic which was started before the operation is continued for at least five days and longer if there is any indication of wound inflammation. It must always be remembered that the elderly patient may be confused and that wandering fingers can interfere with the wound or drains. The suction drains are removed when drainage has ceased, usually three or four days after operation.

On return to the ward the surgeon must have absolute confidence that his operation is secure; that the fracture presents no problem; and the patient may walk forthwith. Therefore it is unnecessary to have more than a simple air-permeable adhesive dressing on the wound: the next day the patient gets up and walks, despite the flasks of the suction drains, which are tied to the walking frame or put in the dressing-gown pocket. This exercise must be part of the routine of the treatment of all such patients; there should be no reservations in the mind of any of those looking after them that early walking has no place or that it is dangerous, because such unspoken anxiety is quickly sensed by the patient. Such worries will not occur if the surgery is of the highest quality.

During this time the relatives are seen by the ward sister and the medical social worker to obtain an accurate assessment of the home and circumstances of the patient. The assessment of the patient in the ward continues by day and particularly by night, during which time any occasional incontinence, confusion, or anxieties become more obvious. If incontinence is present after operation, despite treatment by hourly bladder discipline, the patient is catheterized. It is at this stage that the most ill patients are transferred to the geriatric orthopaedic unit.

GERIATRIC ORTHOPAEDIC UNIT

The geriatric orthopaedic unit is an ordinary ward with a nursing establishment for acute medicine. That the patients are geriatric increases rather than decreases the work load, not because they are in bed but for the very opposite reason: all patients are up and dressed daily.

At the geriatric orthopaedic unit the patient comes under the day to day care of the geriatric physician and his medical staff. The essential feature of the unit is the weekly ward round, at which both physician and surgeon and all members of the team attend; the latter includes the junior medical staff, the ward sister, physiotherapist, occupational therapist, medical social worker, and the ward secretary. The round eliminates paper work among the members of the team with its inherent delay. A comprehensive programme is achieved for all patients, either only for the next week or for the future after the patient's discharge. All patients in the unit are dressed each day and walk. There is no place in a geriatric orthopaedic unit for the bedridden patient. The unit is geared to the patient partaking in the activities of daily living to the best extent possible; his clothes and shoes are therefore kept at the bedside. The occupational therapist instructs and helps in dressing and the other activities of daily living in close co-operation with the physiotherapist who treats—and teaches to walk—each patient as necessary. It is most important to realize that an old person dressed feels "up", whereas in a dressing-gown they feel they should be in bed.

Meanwhile in the acute orthopaedic ward those elderly patients not otherwise ill are discharged home without the necessity of a stay in the unit.

Medical Assessment

The medical assessment of a patient transferred to the geriatric orthopaedic unit has to be comprehensive because the average geriatric patient, especially when frail and senile, usually has several other conditions to be diagnosed and treated. These ailments, including simple anaemia, all impinge on the well-being of the patient and the ability to regain independence. The most common medical conditions seen are cardiovascular disease, urinary infections, renal failure, poor sight, and pulmonary and cerebrovascular disease. Psychiatric disorders occur in about 20% of patients, but these are not necessarily severe and are often sporadic, associated with the sudden admission to hospital with all its fears and strangeness.

Some conditions, such as vertebrobasilar insufficiency may cause the patient to topple backward when walking, and this tendency may be exacerbated by a walking frame, whereas a frame with wheels eliminates the repeated neck flexion and extension which occurs each time the ordinary walking frame is lifted forward.

It a patient complains of persistent pain, particularly after a hip operation, invariably it indicates that all is not well locally and full assessment will find a cause. Never must it be considered that the patient is complaining unduly. Only when the cause has been found and put right can rehabilitation proceed. Similarly some patients fail to progress in walking because the operation is not secure and the feeling of instability caused by this is sufficient to deter progress.

At the weekly ward round, and in all daily routine, the patient must be fully involved; often slight deafness or confusion sets patients apart from a discussion on their wellbeing. If the patient does not understand he may become frightened, confused, and unco-operative. To the enfeebled geriatric patient the separation from home and household goods is very distressing; he needs reassurance not only that he will go home but also that he will not go until he is ready. This restores calm and the wish to progress. There are few old people who, given such assurance, do not want to go home.

Most patients are in the geriatric orthopaedic unit for some three to four weeks; most have then regained their normal level of independence but some may have a medical condition needing further care in a geriatric progressive care ward. A few patients fail to achieve independence and, after careful deliberation, are accepted for long-term stay by the consultant geriatrician. This should never happen because of surgical complications rendering the patient incapable of walking. This again emphasizes the importance of having a surgical technique that gives the lowest possible complication or failure rate.

CARE IN ELECTIVE PROCEDURES

Arthrosis is a pernicious destroyer of independence in the elderly; the condition slowly worsens, and gradually the patient becomes more and more incapacitated until one day he is unable to live at home. It is best to operate long before this stage is reached but many old people still fear a visit to hospital for elective surgery and procrastinate too long. In such enfeebled persons the same methods apply as for the emergency admission and it will readily be appreciated that such patients can have the same programme as the patient with a fracture. But it is still important that the procedure should not keep the patient an unwarrantably long time in bed. Thus an arthroplasty should allow the patient to be up the next day. Prolonged bed rest after such operations can undo all the good in general that the operation has done locally.

The old patient is worried not by the loss of a full range of movement, but by the loss of function commensurate with his general activity in his declining years. It is far better for the patient to achieve independence and a speedy return home than to have a prolonged course of treatment to obtain ranges of movement that he does not need in his normal life. Therefore if the patient can dress; do up shoes laces; walk up stairs; cook; sweep; and get on a bus with no pain or discomfort the operation is highly successful even if movement in the joint concerned is not full. Striving to regain this loss by physiotherapy is unnessary.

SOME GENERAL CONSIDERATIONS

The elderly respond well to operations, which should not be long deferred—though for fractures it is better to rest the patient a few hours (splinted if necessary to control pain) and to operate on the next appropriate list, which should be within twenty-four hours if possible. Whereas in the healthy adult conservative treatment is to be encouraged for such fractures in the femoral or tibial shaft, in the elderly proper and secure internal fixation is always indicated when it can be achieved. The ankle fracture should also be fixed to allow the patient to walk at once, even if in a walking plaster. Even the unstable fracture of the humeral shaft should be internally fixed to allow quick independence.

Fractures of the pelvis and vertebral bodies in old people are almost always stable, and should be treated by early walking. To tell the patient that the backbone has been broken fills them with alarm; instead a careful explanation that there will be some pain because of "heavy bruising of the bone" and advice that, despite this, the general condition will be better if the patient is up allays fear and gives confidence. Mild analgesics are given freely. Once the patient can sit up in bed—usually in a day or two—it is as comfortable to sit in a chair; the latter is no more painful than standing and the patient is quick to achieve walking.

Pathological Fractures and Amputations

Pathological fractures lend themselves to internal fixation. If metastatic deposits in a femur have so weakened the bone that a fracture

L

is imminent, prophylactic intramedullary nailing relieves pain and prevents a catastrophe. Done through the knee joint the operation takes only a few minutes; the hole made between the femoral condyles through which the nail is passed up the shaft is plugged with cement. Other pathological fractures, whether imminent or present, should be dealt with by a similarly active approach, for thereafter radiotherapy is facilitated because there is no pain and no plaster cast. Because the patient may only have a short while to live it is most important that the quality of what little life remains should be satisfactory.

Amputations for vascular disease have a poor prognosis for longevity; the operation is mentally and surgically traumatic, and it may follow an attempt to preserve the limb by vascular surgery. Understandably the old person dreads the loss of a leg and its consequences which are an obvious loss of independence. The sooner therefore that the patient should walk again, the better. Not only this, if the patient can see the new limb—of whatever type—by the bedside at, or soon after, the time of amputation, many anxieties are allayed. At one or two weeks all geriatric amputees should have the means to walk, whether on a sophisticated artificial leg or a simple early walking aid.

CONCLUSIONS

In this short description of geriatric orthopaedics the minutiae of treatment have not been described; nor should they have been, for they are part of the proper practice of medicine. What has been emphasized are the intensive methods needed to give total care to the aged so that they may continue to enjoy an active and independent life. Geriatric patients are dignified in their acceptance of the inevitable end. They do not ask for longevity. They may at times seem anxious, frail, and disheartened; too often this is because they do not understand what is happening. To them it is not existence that matters, but its quality. The aim of all concerned in their treatment must, as in all medicine, be the return of function, but, in the elderly, this is return to independence.

Endocrine Disorders in the Elderly

BY

M. F. GREEN

ANY endocrine abnormality except those affecting menstruation may occur in old people, and many middle-aged people with treated endocrine disease live into old age. Some glandular disorders are common in the elderly (for example, thyroid disease and diabetes mellitus), but only certain hormonal "disease" of old age is the decline in gonadal function—which happens quickly in women at the menopause and more slowly in men in later life. We do not know whether this inevitable ovarian and testicular failure causes ageing of other tissues, though possibly women who have an abnormally early menopause have a shorter life expectation than other women. Probably one reason for the long survival of women compared with men (some five years more, on average) is a protective effect of female hormones from menarche to menopause. Unfortunately we do not have any hormonal therapy which can prevent ageing in either sex by replacement of sex hormones given from middle age onwards, or starting in old age. There is no justification for giving female hormones to men to prevent ageing. The use of oestrogenic hormones in elderly men with prostatic carcinoma is associated with a very substantial risk of thromboembolic disease and fluid retention. Therapy with sex hormones in older people may prove useful in the prevention and treatment of osteoporosis (Nordin[1] has reviewed possible reasons for postmenopausal calcium loss) and help alleviate arthritic and inflammatory conditions by interfering with prostaglandin synthesis. These are fascinating speculations but it is much more important to discuss the problems of diagnosing, investigating, and treating "classical" endocrine syndromes affecting old people.

Endocrine syndromes may present at any age with a florid picture of hyperactivity (for example, exophthalmic thyrotoxicosis) or hypoactivity (for example, hypopituitarism). Nevertheless, these are rare in very old people, probably because of the way endocrine dysfunction tends to have widespread and non-specific effects, the modifying effects of other accumulated pathologies, and multiple prescribing. The second and third factors are very common in old age and both modify target-organ response and laboratory tests. Our inpatients have an average of almost one endocrine "problem" each, classifying problems as proved endocrine diseases and abnormal endocrine function tests without apparent disease. Over half are receiving three or more

L*

drugs. The problems of interpreting the results of abnormal laboratory tests in the elderly are very great, and we may also miss people with occult disease but apparently normal tests. Neoplastic disease is common in old age and may be associated with a whole range of endocrine syndromes (which are often atypical), so that we may also be missing endocrine problems associated with malignancies.

It is difficult to decide whether all or many old people should be subjected to some form of biochemical screening. Hospital surveys have shown a high incidence of disorders affecting pancreatic and thyroidal function, and calcium and electrolyte balance. In deciding on the need for screening the following important points should be remembered:

(1) Great clinical skill may be needed to identify all the different medical problems affecting an old person.

(2) Endocrine disease is common in old age, can be lethal, and may be easy to treat once diagnosed.

(3) There are practical and semantic difficulties in the concept of a "normal" range for biochemical values in old age—abnormal results are common but do not always imply endocrine disease.

(4) Side effects of any treatment should be balanced against the complications of the disease being treated with even more care than in younger people. This is particularly important when the diagnosis of the disease may be difficult, and any drug therapy may overload an elderly recipient's mental capabilities and metabolizing and clearance systems.

DIABETES MELLITUS

About a quarter of the population over 75 have abnormal (diabetic) glucose tolerance tests.[3] It is often difficult and usually unnecessary to perform a standard test in old people, and the diagnosis can often be made from a single blood sugar estimation and the clinical features. A clearly raised random, fasting, or two hour postprandial value may be diagnostic. It has been suggested[4] that the most practical approach is to regard a random level of more than 165 mg/100 ml as an indication for a GTT, if not proof in its own right. Urine testing may not always reveal glycosuria in elderly people with hyperglycaemia because of the general decline of glomerular filtration rate and rise in renal glucose threshold. Blood-glucose estimation should be obtained in emergencies if possible, but Dextrostix or Reflectance-meter-Dextrostix measurement may help in making rapid clinical decisions, particularly in suspected hypoglycaemia.

Severe hyperglycaemia may develop rapidly for the first time at any age, but most older diabetics have a mild disturbance of carbohydrate metabolism. Complications of the disease and of treatment (see table) are usually more important than hyperglycaemia. The problem is to decide what antidiabetic treatment (if any) apart from that demanded by diabetic coma will minimize or prevent the associated diseases. Energetic treatment may have serious hazards, and the long-term benefits of sulphonylureas have been doubted, with evidence from an American survey[5] [6] conflicting with opinion from other parts of the world.

Complications of Diabetes Mellitus and of its Treatment

Mechanism or Target Organ	Effect
Hyperglycaemia	Keto-acidotic coma Hyperosmolar non-ketotic coma
Atherosclerosis	Cerebral, coronary, renal, mesenteric thrombosis Peripheral vessels
Kidney	Infections, nephrosis, renal failure
Eyes	Cataracts Diabetic and atherosclerotic retinopathy
Nerves	Autonomic neuropathy (postural hypotension, diarrhoea) Sensory neuropathy (painless ulceration of feet) Amyotrophy (affecting legs)
Infections	Skin (especially of feet and flexures), chest, renal
Treatment	Hypoglycaemia (neuroglycopenia) Long-term morbidity of oral agents

Keto-acidosis may develop for the first time in very old people. They tend to succumb rapidly to metabolic disturbances and infections, which may be the cause of or the consequence of deterioration. Abdominal pain may be a striking feature (as well as polydipsia, polyuria, dehydration, etc.), and is also common in non-ketotic hyperosmolar coma. This may occur at any age,[7] but is more frequent in older age groups, and often develops in people not previously known to be diabetic. Urine testing and blood-sugar measurements are therefore indicated in confused or comatose elderly people particularly if they are dehydrated and have complained previously of thirst, polyuria, and abdominal pain.

Management

If an older person has diabetes requiring treatment, some instruction about the disease should be given if possible (and to relatives and friends where necessary); this should explain the significance of urine testing and of treatment prescribed. Dietary advice may be difficult to follow even when carefully explained, and an additional problem in the elderly is that carbohydrate-rich diets are usually cheap and well-wishers may offer tempting sugary foods. It is distressingly common to find oral agents and insulin prescribed for old people who have not been told about the possible side effects. When urine tests are performed, negative results in spite of underlying hyperglycaemia are common, which may protect old people from over-enthusiastic treatment. It may be necessary to accept random blood sugar levels of 150–200 mg/100 ml as satisfactory, and even higher levels are sometimes tolerated remarkably well.

The principles of treatment are the same at any age:

Diet

Carbohydrate intake should be restricted if possible (for example, 100–120 g/day in a small elderly woman), as should total calories in the obese. Dietary advice is still important for those on tablets and insulin.

Oral Antidiabetic Agents

Oral antidiabetic drugs are cumulative and may cause severe prolonged hypoglycaemia in the elderly, who usually require smaller doses than younger diabetics. Other side effects include gastrointestinal upsets, rashes, and jaundice. Tolbutamide (up to 0·5 g thrice daily), and chlorpropamide (100 to 350 mg/day) are still the most useful, and may be supplemented with a biguanide especially in the obese (but gastrointestinal side effects are common).

Insulin

More than one injection a day should be avoided if possible, by using Insulin Zinc (Lente) or by giving soluble and protamine zinc insulin (PZI) injections at the same time. A sliding scale of insulin dosage is indicated to cover illnesses and operations, but as it only prevents trouble by frequent monitoring of past events, the aim should be an early return to insulin once a day. It is often possible to stop insulin entirely after concurrent illness is treated. Another person will need to inject insulin if the diabetic is confused or has poor sight.

Hyperglycaemia

A general practitioner may be able to identify and reverse deteriorating control in an elderly diabetic at home, but precoma and coma are medical emergencies. Both ketotic and hyperosmolar forms require intensive hospital care, with frequent biochemical estimations, and specific treatment for precipitating causes such as chest and urine infections. The mortality rate is well above the 10% described for younger patients,[8] even if a geriatric or medical ward is used to managing such patients.

Hypoglycaemia

Hypoglycaemia may not be obvious and can cause confusion or headache, as well as shivering, sweating, and vasoconstriction. These attacks may occur at any time of the day or night. Neuroglycopenia is a serious hazard and may rapidly cause severe and permanent brain damage. If prevention by cautious drug therapy and patient education has failed, rapid correction of a low blood sugar is imperative. Intravenous glucose is effective but messy to handle, and improvement may not be so rapid as with glucagon. This can be given parenterally (and by a nurse) in a dose of 0·25 mg, and should be in a general practitioner's emergency bag. Treatment with glucagon or glucose is usually justified in suspected but non-proved cases of hypoglycaemia in the elderly and failure to improve does not necessarily disprove the diagnosis. Recovery should be followed with oral carbohydrate, and long-term measures to prevent recurrence.

Associated Diseases

Disease associated with diabetes read like a catalogue of geriatric medicine (see table), and are usually more important than the diabetes. Some aggravate pre-existing diabetes or lead to its discovery—for example, chest and urinary infections. Simple measures to control some of these diseases may be very effective, including care of the skin, sensible footwear, and chiropody. Conservative or extensive surgery for infections, neuropathies, and arteriopathies of the feet and legs may be justified, even in very old people.

Most blind people are elderly.[9] Diabetic retinopathy and cataracts in a diabetic are common causes of blindness. Like many of the "associated" diseases, cataract tends to develop at a younger age and progress more rapidly in diabetics than in non-diabetics. Cataract extraction should always be considered even in a severe elderly diabetic, and may make a dramatic difference to life, including a return to independence for urine testing and insulin administration. Registration of those with partial or no sight is financially helpful, though it may be difficult to find suitable local authority accommodation once an elderly person has been registered.

The main aims of treatment in elderly diabetics are to avoid hypoglycaemia and severe hyperglycaemia, to reduce gross obesity, and to minimize the development and progression of associated diseases.

THYROID DISEASE

Myxoedema, thyrotoxicosis, and symptoms and signs which may be due to thyroid disease are common in old age and several lesions may contribute to one or more of the clinical features in ill old people. This is particularly true of thyroid dysfunction—for example, confusion, anaemia, constipation, and ischaemic heart disease may coexist with (and hide) hypothyroidism, or be caused by it. Similarly thyrotoxicosis may contribute to confusion, diarrhoea, and congestive cardiac failure. Both may develop insidiously and be so atypical that even a doctor with a high index of suspicion can miss the diagnosis: it has happened that a thyrotoxic old lady has been suspected initially of being myxoedematous.

These diagnostic problems and the serious complications of treatment justify asking for laboratory confirmation of suspected thyroid disease in old age.

Over 5% of our geriatric admissions have thyroid disease and many more have abnormal thyroid function tests. Abnormal tests are often caused by changes in plasma proteins,[10] which are common in old age, in ill people, and may be caused by drugs interfering with protein-binding. X-ray media and drugs many also affect tests by iodide contamination and other mechanisms. Present evidence suggests that all old people admitted to hospital, and any old person at home who is suspected of having thyroid disease, should have thyroid function tests carried out. This usually means at least two in-vitro tests (in addition to any other "screening" tests for other occult but common pathologies) such as protein-bound-iodine (PBI) and tri-iodothyronine (T-3) resin uptake, serum T-3 and thyroxine (T-4), free thyroxine index (FTI) or effective thyroxine ratio (ETR), or any combination offered by the laboratory. The aim is to minimize conflicting evidence from abnormal tests and the clinical picture. It may still be necessary to ask for in-vivo test such as thyroidal gland uptake.

Assessment of target organ function is rarely helpful in diagnosing thyroid dysfunction in old age, as it may be abnormal for other reasons (for example, weight, pulse, serum cholesterol, ECG) or difficult to elicit (for example, tendon reflex relaxation time). Such assessment may be more useful in monitoring the response to treatment, particularly when the results of investigations have been conflicting and treatment has been started mainly on clinical grounds.

Hypothyroidism

The prevalence of hypothyroidism in the aged is uncertain. Preliminary analysis of thyroid function tests in volunteers taking part in a survey in Camden (part of a National Hypothermia Study[11]) has shown that over 4% had hypothyroid results. The sample was not random, but the subjects were all living at home and relatively fit so this figure may be an underestimate.

Many doctors will have seen cold, bloated, constipated, and apathetic old women with myxoedema who have responded dramatically to replacement therapy. Some of these patients (and others with less obvious but proven hypothyroidism) die soon after starting treatment. This may be because other lesions have taken their toll, but cardiac function in the elderly is particularly vulnerable to excessive and too rapid thyroxine replacement. Treatment must therefore be based on a combination of clinical acumen and laboratory confirmation, and the response to treatment monitored very carefully. Iatrogenically-induced myxoedema has been recommended to alleviate angina, but cardiac (and respiratory) function is improved after treating hypothyroidism.[12] Cautious but effective treatment is therefore justified in myxoedematous patients with ischaemic heart disease.

Clinical suspicion of thyroid lack should be aroused by the presence of a goitre or thyroidectomy scar, a history of thyroid treatment, a family history of thyroid disease, and the finding of a slow pulse or delayed relaxation of tendon reflexes. Cold intolerance, dry skin, croaky voice, deafness, rheumatism, ataxia, constipation, and confusion are common but non-specific features. A past history of antithyroid treatment is particularly significant. The risk of developing hypothyroidism after both radio-iodine and surgical treatment of thyrotoxicosis is so high[13][14] that such patients should be followed up for life. A computer-based hospital/general-practitioner system has been developed in Aberdeen for this purpose.[15] It has also been suggested[16] that treatment is often discontinued or inadequate in myxoedematous patients.

There is no justification for replacement therapy with anything other than L-thyroxine (LT-4).

Thyroid extract, L-tri-iodothyronine (LT-3), and LT-4/LT-3 mixtures have no advantage apart from treating hypothermia caused by hypothyroidism with rapidly acting LT-3. Myxoedema is a rare cause of hypothermia (which has been discussed more fully in another article), but the clinical features and results of tests done while the patient is hypothermic may falsely suggest myxoedema.

LT-4 treatment should be started cautiously in the elderly. An initial daily dose of 0·05 mg will produce its maximum effect after one or two weeks, when a full reassessment of the clinical state and target-organ function will usually justify a cautious increase in the daily dose by 0·025 or 0·05 mg. Further small increments may be introduced at similar intervals, and few old people need more than

0·2 mg a day to restore euthyroidism. Some seem to need as much as 0·5 or 0·6 mg of LT-4 a day but should reach this dose only after a long period of close hospital and general-practitioner liaison. If thyroid-stimulating-hormone (TSH) assay becomes widely available and less controversial it may help judge the adequacy of LT-4 treatment. In spite of apparently adequate therapy the symptoms and signs may not improve on LT-4—the mental state may remain impaired and constipation and heart failure persist—and a raised TSH level would then justify increasing the dose.

Angina and heart failure may get worse during the initial stages of treatment, and even heart attacks and sudden death may occur in elderly patients. If heart disease worsens at the start of treatment a β-adrenergic blocking agent may be added to the LT-4. Propanolol is used (for example, at a dose of 5–10 mg thrice daily) but may aggravate heart failure and hypotension so that the more cardioselective practolol may be preferable.

Hyperthyroidism

All the cases of thyrotoxicosis admitted to a geriatric unit were "atypical",[17] and were 2% of all admissions. Loss of weight, muscle weakness, apathy, and cardiac abnormalities tend to dominate the clinical picture in old people. A basic rule in the elderly is that more than one disease may be causing the same problem. Cardiac failure, even with clear evidence of ischaemic heart disease, may be refractory to treatment because of hyperthyroidism. Absence of atrial fibrillation would militate against the diagnosis as this is so very common in old people with heart disease and with thyrotoxicosis.

The results of thyroid function tests in the elderly may be slightly less confusing in suspected hyperthyroidism than in myxoedema, and studies of radio-iodine uptake by the thyroid gland may be more useful. The likelihood that the recently described syndrome of T-3 thyrotoxicosis may cause disease in very old people has not yet been confirmed, but may be the reason for a clinical suspicion of hyperthyroidism being negated by apparently normal test results.

The great risk of hypothyroidism after both surgical and radio-iodine treatment of thyrotoxicosis has been mentioned. The incidence of hypothyroidism is already high one year after treatment, with a continuing rise in the risk with each subsequent year. Though radio-iodine is an easy treatment which can be given to outpatients, it does not usually bring a hyperactive thyroid under control for some months. Antithyroid drugs are therefore the treatment of first choice in old people and carbimazole is the most widely used drug in the UK. An average starting dose of 15 mg thrice daily may be reduced to 5–10 mg thrice daily after some months. Rashes and blood dyscrasias

are relatively uncommon side effects. β-adrenergic blockers (see hypothyroidism) may be useful particularly in patients with tachycardia,
and we have successfully controlled elderly thyrotoxics on propanolol
alone. Any antithyroid drug should be reviewed regularly, and can be
discontinued when the disease remits, which is usually between one
and two years after the onset.

CALCIUM AND ELECTROLYTES

Diseases affecting calcium and electrolyte balance, and abnormal
values obtained in biochemical screening, are common in old people.
They are discussed in detail in other papers in this series, but endocrine
factors are often important.

Abnormally high and low calcium values are often found in elderly
patients admitted to hospital. Hypercalcaemia is often associated with
neoplastic disease (of bronchus, breast, prostate and rarely colon)
due to bony metastases or "ectopic" parathormone production by the
tumour. This and other ectopic hormone syndromes associated with
carcinoma may occur in very old people. They may cause gross biochemical disturbances and illnesses such as hypercalcaemia with
gastrointestinal upset and renal damage, and oversecretion of adreno-
corticotrophic hormone with all the hazards of Cushing's syndrome
(especially weakness and confusion due to potassium and chloride loss).
Hyperparathyroidism may cause mental impairment but it is depress-
ingly unrewarding to search for it and for other biochemical causes of
dementia (such as myxoedema or vitamin B_{12} deficiency). Hypercalcaemia is also a real risk of excessive vitamin D treatment of osteomalacia.

Paget's Disease

The recently discovered hormone thyrocalcitonin has been recommended to treat Paget's disease[18] and osteoporosis, because of its action in
inhibiting bone resorption. Its use in both diseases is rather empirical
because there is no evidence that it is remedying a deficiency state.
Response is difficult to monitor because both diseases tend to have been
present for a long time before diagnosis, and the only abnormality
of calcium biochemistry is a raised alkaline phosphatase in Paget's
disease and sometimes a slightly raised alkaline phosphatase in osteoporosis immediately after a fracture.

Aldosterone

Hyperaldosteronism may occur in old people with congestive
cardiac failure and hepatic and renal disease, and causes salt and water
retention. An aldosterone anatagonist (for example, spironolactone

25 mg thrice daily) may be useful in clearing resistant oedema but may have to be added to an already complicated drug regimen and take some two to three weeks to produce its maximum effect. Ankle oedema in the elderly is common, and it is often unnecessary to abolish it by obsessional treatment even if other signs of heart failure are present.

Antidiuretic Hormone

Secretion of antidiuretic hormone may be inappropriately increased in several conditions affecting the elderly—such as carcinoma of the bronchus, pneumonia, and hypothyroidism. The effect is to produce a low serum osmolality due to water retention and sodium loss. This causes vague symptoms of weakness, loss of appetite, confusion, and eventually death. Treatment may be difficult but should be as energetic as possible as the symptoms may be so unpleasant. Treatment of underlying conditions, and by water restriction, should be monitored biochemically.

ADRENAL FUNCTION

Some abnormalities of adrenal function tests have been described in elderly people without endocrine disease[19], but there is no evidence of any decline in adrenal cortical or medullary function in old age. Corticosteroids may be indicated in the treatment of specific diseases such as rheumatoid arthritis. They may also be used in larger non-physiological doses in "shocked" patients. The mineralocorticoid $\propto$-fludrocortisone is sometimes helpful in treating postural hypotension, though getting up slowly, "heavy-duty" tights, and salt supplements are more useful.

GONADAL FUNCTION

One important effect of the decline in gonadal function in old age is that changes in secondary sexual characteristics may cause mild or serious disability (for example, "senile" vaginitis or leukoplakia) and/or reduce sexual activity in elderly couples who might otherwise have continued a more physical relationship. Of course, older people are influenced by their own and society's emotional attitudes, which have tended to encourage a reduction in the physical aspects of sexual relationships. Nevertheless, strong physical and mental links may persist into extremely old age. One consequence is the way the survivor of a very long partnership often dies soon after the other. It is difficult to make any specific recommendantion regarding replacement therapy. Short and long-term sex-hormone therapy have serious hazards when given parenterally but they occasionally help improve incontinence. Topical applications of an oestrogen cream may help so-called "senile" vaginitis (the patient is not really senile—she is old and has a medical problem). Bleeding may be a problem with such creams, and topical corticosteroids may be effective, though they too have side effects.

CONCLUSIONS

There is no evidence that hormone supplements or hormonal ablation can improve the health or life-expectation of old people, unless indicated to treat a specific endocrine disease. Endocrine diseases are common in old age and may often be atypical in their presentation. Great skill may be needed in their diagnosis and management.

REFERENCES

[1] Nordin, B. E. C., *British Medical Journal*, 1971, **1**, 571.
[2] McKeown, F., *Pathology of the Aged*. London, Butterworths, 1965.
[3] Butterfield, W. J. H., *Proceedings of the Royal Society of Medicine*, 1964, **57**, 196.
[4] Denham, M. J., *Age and Ageing*, **1**, 55.
[5] University Group Diabetics Program, *Diabetics*, 1970, **19**, *Supplement*, **2**, 747.
[6] University Group Diabetes Program, *Journal of the American Medical Association*, 1971, **217**, 777.
[7] Walde, D., Whelton, M. J., and Havard, C. W. H., *British Medical Journal*, 1971, **1**, 85.
[8] Hockaday, T. D. R., and Alberti, K. G. M. M., *British Journal of Hospital Medicine*, 1972, **7**, 183.
[9] Sorsby, A., *Health Trends*, 1973, **5**, 7.
[10] Jefferys, P. M., Farran, H. E. A., Hoffenberg, R., Fraser, P. M., and Hodkinson, H. M., *Lancet*, 1972, **2**, 974.
[11] Fox, R. H., Woodward, P. M., Exton-Smith, A. N., Green, M. F., Donnison, D. V., and Wicks, M. H., *British Medical Journal*, 1973, **1**, 200.
[12] Burack, R., Edwards, R. H. T., Green, M. F., and Jones, N. L., *Journal of Pharmacology and Experimental Therapeutics*, 1971, **1**, 212.
[13] Green, M., and Wilson, G. M., *British Medical Journal*, 1964, **1**, 1005.
[14] Michie, E., Pegg, C. A. S., and Bewsher, P. D., *British Medical Journal*, 1972, **1**, 13.
[15] Hedley, A. J., Flemming, C. J., Chesters, M. I., Michie, W., and Crooks, J., *British Medical Journal*, 1970, **1**, 519.
[16] Hedley, A. J., *Practitioner*, 1972, **208**, 349.
[17] Jefferys, P. M., *Age and Ageing*, 1972, **1**, 33.
[18] Woodhouse, M. J. Y., *et al.*, *Lancet*, 1972, **2**, 1139.
[19] Green, M. F., and Friedman, M., *Gerontologia Clinica*, 1968, **10**, 334.

INDEX